DATE DUE

MY ~~0 9~~			
~~OE 7 '98~~			
~~AP 27 '00~~			
~~MY 1 9'00~~			
~~FE 1 3 '02~~			
~~OE 3'03~~			
~~MY 1 0 '06~~			

DEMCO 38-296

The Changing Health Care Marketplace

The Changing Health Care Marketplace

Private Ventures, Public Interests

Walter A. Zelman

Jossey-Bass Publishers • San Francisco

Substantial discounts on bulk quantities of Jossey-Bass books are available to corporations, professional associations, and other organizations. For details and discount information, contact the special sales department at Jossey-Bass Inc., Publishers (415) 433–1740; Fax (800) 605–2665.

For sales outside the United States, please contact your local Simon & Schuster International Office.

TCF Manufactured in the United States of America on Lyons Falls Pathfinder Tradebook. This paper is acid-free and 100 percent totally chlorine-free.

Library of Congress Cataloging-in-Publication Data

Zelman, Walter A.
  The changing health care marketplace : private ventures, public interests / Walter A. Zelman. — 1st ed.
      p. cm.
  Includes bibliographical references and index.
  ISBN 0–7879–0252–7 (cloth: acid-free paper)
  1. Managed care plans (Medical care)—United States. 2. Integrated delivery of health care—United States. 3. Medical policy—United States. I. Title.
RA410.53.Z45 1996
362.1'0973—dc20   96–9984
                                                           CIP

HB Printing 10 9 8 7 6 5 4 3 2 1   FIRST EDITION

Contents

For Georgia and Rebecca
And all those for whom efficient private
health care markets will not be enough

Preface

A few months ago, in the middle of a presentation on health care trends and new health care partnerships I was asked: "Walter, what does all this mean for people?"

The inquiry was premature. In fact, the second half of my presentation was going to address exactly that question. Still, the question was a jarring one. Today, amid the great sweep of health care marketplace change—some of which may not be as sweeping as first appears to be the case—it is easy to get lost in the details of who's partnering or competing with whom, what markets are changing fastest, what risk-sharing strategies are being invoked where, and so on.

The process and extent of change, in short, is fascinating in and of itself. It's hardly surprising, then, that the first question usually asked is What's going on?—not, What does it mean? In many cases, the second question doesn't even get asked. When the meaning question is asked, the analysis is likely to focus on what change may mean for those directly and economically involved—the insurers, hospitals, physicians, and others engaged in the organizing, purchasing, selling, or delivery of health care services. Indeed, until quite recently at least, the greatest quantity of analysis—sometimes the only analysis—of market change came from those serving as consultants to the major actors and from professional journals whose readers are those same actors. Not surprisingly, such analysis focuses on the impact of change for those actors and on what those actors might do to improve their positioning in the emerging marketplace.

Taking something of a back seat in all this is the subject area my questioner was raising: "What does all this mean for people?" And, one might add, for public policy.

Thus, this book has two purposes. First, it defines and explores some of the origins and key attributes of current marketplace change—especially the formation of new, sometimes uneasy partnerships among physicians, hospitals, and health plans. Second, it analyzes the implications of those changes for public interests and public policy.

The second purpose, especially, may seem a bit audacious. If there is great debate (and, I might add, often great distortion) as to what is actually going on in the health care marketplace, how can one propose what to do about it? Probably, one can't. But one can begin to raise questions and to anticipate effects that policy makers will need to eventually—and in some cases quickly—address.

Overview of Contents

Part One, which includes Chapters One and Two, outlines the rise of managed care and the growth of prepayment, risk-sharing strategies (including capitation, withholds, and bonuses) that are central to its cost containment goals. Trends are outlined and explored, as are the long-term prospects that managed care and various risk-sharing strategies can reduce health care costs and premiums while maintaining if not improving quality of care delivered.

Part Two focuses on the emerging partnerships—among physicians, hospitals, and insurers—that the rise of managed care and its payment strategies may be fostering. Chapter Three suggests these partnerships may be viewed largely as means to secure access to and control over the managed care premium dollar and to secure positioning in the organized delivery systems (ODSs) that most anticipate will dominate health care delivery in the near future.

Chapter Four reviews trends in consolidation within each sector—insurers with insurers, hospitals with hospitals, and physicians with physicians. Such consolidation, it appears, is generally the first step in new partnership activity. Chapter Five reviews relationships among the three sectors, focusing especially on the efforts of all, clearly critical in the managed care era, to secure the services and commitment of primary care physicians. Chapter Six reviews the rise—modest as it sometimes may be—of the ODS and the many forms such systems may take. An effort is also made to assess the assets and liabilities of the major actors in organizing and leading these systems.

Part Three focuses on implications for the general public and for public policy of the rise of managed care and risk-sharing strategies, as well as of the new partnerships and delivery system organizations. Chapter Seven briefly reviews one critical cause of the failure of the Clinton administration's health care reform effort, but emphasizes that while reform may have died, all the issues of health care policy remain. The analysis then goes on to underscore the need to keep the marketplace competitive, especially in the absence of direct government intervention, and what policy makers may want, or not want, to do in pursuit of that goal.

Chapter Eight reviews the potential for marketplace change to affect the value of health care purchases—either by lowering the price of that care or by raising its quality. The potential to do both (especially to lower price) is present. However, when it comes to raising quality, the question of whether the ultimate impact of market forces and changes is much more uncertain. Chapter Nine reviews how consumers might best be served, or in some cases protected, under the new paradigm of less may be better. Chapter Ten looks at those roles—care for the uninsured, provisions for a safety net, care for the elderly and the poor, and so on—that have long been public responsibilities. It is in this realm that some of the greatest policy concerns may arise, as marketplace forces (and potential government actions) put stress on the indirect subsidies that have supported the safety net, without replacing those indirect subsidies with direct subsidies.

Methodological Notes

It's never easy to study change while it is occurring.

The Problem of Terminology

As might be expected, as organizations change and as hybrids emerge, terminology fails to keep pace. Today this is most evident in the definitions of health maintenance organization (HMO) forms. The traditional breakdown of HMOs into staff, group, network, and independent practice association (IPA) models is fast losing its value. Increasing numbers of HMOs offer several types of plans, making it more difficult to classify them. Additionally, the plans offered by HMOs are, increasingly, hybrids of one or more types. The not surprising net result is that comparisons between HMO types are often problematic, at best. (The issue of merging forms of HMOs is discussed in greater detail in Chapter One.)

Another issue of terminology relates to the terms *insurer, managed care organization (MCO), HMO,* and *health plan,* which often seem to be used interchangeably in the literature. In this book, *insurer* refers to the broadest category, including organizations offering insurance in any form. *MCO* denotes insurers offering managed care plans—such as preferred provider organizations (PPOs) or health maintenance organizations. I use *HMO* to identify prepaid, fixed-price managed care arrangements. *Health plan* means any particular offering or option—a PPO, a point-of-service (POS) plan, a high or low option plan, or even an IPA model HMO—marketed by an insurer, which may be offering many such plans.

Gathering Information on Market Change

At conferences focused on changing health care markets today, the same phrases and concerns are voiced repeatedly. "If you've seen one PHO, you've seen one PHO." "I spent eight months collecting data only to discover it was out of date." "I need to change the slides in my presentation at least monthly."

In other words, change appears to be occurring (it isn't always) at such a dramatic pace that research involving the systematic collection and analysis of data is sometimes focused on organizations or markets that are changing rapidly or may no longer exist. If market change is to be understood or even attempted, then, such systematic research must be buttressed by case studies and even anecdote.

Information and data for this book were collected from five primary sources:

1. Rigorous, systematic research that is publicly available, and some that is not fully available to the public.
2. Research on trends, and analysis of trends, undertaken by trade associations and consulting firms—for example, the American Hospital Association, the American Medical Association, the Group Health Association of America, Foster Hig-

gins, and KPMG Peat Marwick and Associates. Much of this research is based on surveys that entail sampling limitations.

3. Reports from periodicals and newspapers, most of which are anecdotal in nature.

4. Published (and sometimes unpublished) articles and analysis by health policy analysts, consultants, lawyers, government officials, and interest group representatives.

5. A series of over sixty interviews with experts—researchers, analysts, and practitioners—that I conducted between December 1994 and January 1996. Information obtained in these interviews was particularly valuable in assessing the actual state of marketplace developments and the potential impact of those developments on specific market sectors, organizations, professional groups, or the general public. A partial list of interviewees is included in the Appendix.

One Caveat

Given the pace of change, and the need to rely on secondary sources, I presume that this book includes errors—certainly of judgment, and perhaps even of fact. A reported merger may not have taken place; in fact, it may never have gotten off the ground. An unpublished study and even some published ones might have been seriously flawed.

The effort to check all information presented in this book in a timely fashion was considerable; checking that information again two months later has proved impossible.

Therefore, I wish to apologize in advance to any organizations or individuals about which or whom any inaccurate information may be presented.

Acknowledgments

I wish to thank the individuals—primarily consultants, lawyers, practitioners, academics, policy analysts, and so on—who submitted to lengthy interviews and who offered an unending wealth of insights to the nature of current market changes and to the potential impact of that change. In particular, I wish to thank Jacque Sokolov, Lynn Etheredge, and researchers at the Group Health Association of

America and the Advisory Board Company for their time, insights, and research assistance. Invaluable assistance was also provided by representatives of the following organizations: the American Hospital Association, especially Ellen Pryga; the American Medical Association, especially Edward Hirshfeld; the American Group Practice Association, especially Donald Fisher and M. Kathleen Kenyon; and the Medical Group Management Association, especially David Gans. Professors Harold S. Luft and Stephen M. Shortell and attorney Peter Grant offered valuable analysis and reviewed early drafts. Professor Roice Luke of Virginia Commonwealth University was particularly generous in sharing research findings.

The Agency for Health Care Policy and Research provided research support for the project. Librarian Renee McCullough was extremely helpful in locating and providing the most up-to-date research on relevant issues.

Finally, I want to thank my personal and primary in-house physician, Dr. Georgia Goldfarb, who kept reminding me that, ultimately, the delivery of high-quality health care will not depend on the establishment of larger and more complex administrative and financial structures. Rather, it will depend on the skills, dedication, and coordination that individuals and teams—perhaps working in more sophisticated and more supportive systems—can bring to the task.

Washington, D.C.   WALTER A. ZELMAN
March 1996

The Author

WALTER A. ZELMAN is a health policy analyst who worked in the White House during the recent health care reform effort. He earned his B.A. degree (1965) in political science from the University of Michigan and the London School of Economics and both his M.A. degree (1966) in international relations and his Ph.D. degree (1971) in American politics from the University of California, Los Angeles.

After a few years of teaching in Southern California colleges and universities, Zelman left the teaching of politics for more activist endeavors. For twelve years, he served as the executive director of California Common Cause, a public interest group focusing on political reform issues, especially campaign financing and government ethics. During the 1980s, Zelman broadened the agenda to include a series of consumer protection organizations' efforts, especially in the field of insurance. He was widely regarded as a leader in the California consumer and political reform communities and published many articles on California government and politics.

In 1989, he left Common Cause to run for the office of California State Insurance Commissioner. While receiving endorsements of consumer leaders and editorial boards, Zelman lost in a primary race to John Garamendi, who went on to win the general election. In 1991, Garamendi hired Zelman as special deputy for health insurance. In that role, Zelman led a special commission in an effort to formulate a new health care reform proposal for California. The result, *California Health Care in the 21st Century,* advocated achievement of universal health care via vigorous competition between private health care organizations.

The proposal won national recognition as a unique blend of reform approaches. It attracted the interest of, among others,

Presidential candidate Bill Clinton. In January 1993, Zelman was invited to work on the White House's health care reform effort. In that capacity, he helped to develop the Clinton administration's reform proposal and to explain its rationale to interest groups and the general public.

Since leaving the White House in late 1994, Zelman has researched changes in the health care marketplace and the policy implications of those changes.

The Changing
Health Care
Marketplace

Prologue

Looking back, it all seems to have been pretty inevitable. Perhaps it was impossible to predict the forms change would take, or what match might set the tinder on fire. The precise timing of change was also unclear. It could have happened a few years earlier, or even a few years later. And the pace and impact of change were unpredictable—they still are.

But the coming of change, even major change, was inevitable. The health care marketplace could not forever sustain double-digit increases in health care premiums.

If the politician runs for election on a platform of "Jobs, jobs, and jobs," by the late 1980s the issue in health care was "Costs, costs, and costs."

Labor disputes were no longer about increasing wages; they were about reducing health care benefits. Study after study was being published proclaiming U.S. health care costs to be higher than any competitor nation (a fact not lost on those competing in the world marketplace) with overall quality of care not demonstrably any better. Other studies were revealing that some communities had far greater health care costs and medical intervention rates than others, but were producing no higher quality of care.

Small and lower-wage employers found the situation increasingly untenable, and many responded by reducing coverage, demanding that employees pay a larger share of rising premiums, or by dropping insurance altogether. The numbers of the uninsured climbed.

Larger employers sought refuge in self-insurance and the greater market leverage granted by size. But by the end of the 1980s, while many of their health care managers had learned a great deal about health care delivery and purchasing (and that knowledge would prove to be important), one of the things they were learning was that they were rather ineffective at controlling health care costs.

1

To some, managed care plans, especially health maintenance organizations (HMOs), appeared to hold an answer. As prepaid plans, they provided incentives for controlling costs and an alternative to the cost-unconscious fee-for-service system in which doing more—and often charging more—was rewarded with higher provider revenues and profits.

But in the late 1980s, HMOs still maintained but a small share of the market. About thirty-five million individuals were in HMOs in 1989 (Group Health Association of America, 1995a), and HMOs had achieved significant penetration levels in only a few major markets. At the end of 1991, only four states—California, Massachusetts, Minnesota, and Oregon—and the District of Columbia had more than 25 percent of their populations in HMOs (Group Health Association of America, 1992). With a nationwide penetration rate of just 15 percent, most HMOs, it seemed, were not yet competing against each other, but against fee-for-service plans. The phrase often used to describe such competition was *shadow pricing*, in which HMOs would offer more benefits and somewhat lower (but not lower than necessary) premiums than fee-for-service plans.

In the search for solutions, Democrats and liberals emphasized universal coverage (and the mandates needed to get there) and leaned toward regulatory solutions in which government rate setting would play a major role, as in Canada or Medicare. With a few exceptions, Republicans offered much less—not perhaps because they saw no problem, but because they weren't prepared to advocate significant levels of government intervention to address the problem. With Republicans in the White House and huge blocks of interest groups wary of regulatory approaches, Democratic solutions had little hope. Republican solutions, such as they were, were generally too modest to attract enough interest in the Democratic-dominated Congress. As a result, politics offered stalemate, rather than an answer—nor did it offer even a serious threat of action, which, as would soon prove to be the case, might have been enough to get market change started.

The Rise and Fall, and Rise, of Reform

But in the early 1990s, several developments occurred that may have set the stage and opened the door to widespread marketplace change.

First, just as costs and premiums seemed to be rising out of control, managed care organizations (MCOs) appeared to be getting some control over them. Partly as a result of MCOs beginning to compete against each other, and partly as a result of employer pressures, rates of increase in premiums in MCOs began to fall. Moreover, differences in premium costs between MCOs and fee-for-service plans began to expand.

Many, including some of the nation's leading health economists, remained unconvinced that managed care could really lower costs, especially if lower costs meant a consistent slowing in the rate of growth in these costs. But employers saw little need to wait for the historical verdict. The result was a modest stampede toward managed care. Within just six years, between 1988 and 1994, the proportion of the population with employer-sponsored insurance who were in MCOs rose from 29 percent to 70 percent (Samuelson, 1995).

The rising numbers in MCOs represented substantial change. By the end of 1994, over fifty million people were enrolled in HMOs. But just as important was the way those rising numbers fueled further competition between MCOs. In seventeen states, including most of the most populous states, over 20 percent of individuals were now in HMOs, and the national HMO market share stood at just under 20 percent (Group Health Association of America, 1995a). In an effort to lower premiums and appeal to more employers, organizers of MCOs began to increase pressure on providers to improve efficiency and to lower utilization and costs. As they did so, they in effect became allies of the demand side, shifting the balance that, in the health care marketplace, had long favored the supply side.

As for providers, they began feeling a sudden need to be part of networks, HMOs, or other organizations that seemed to increasingly control the health care revenue stream. An uneasy search for new partners was on.

Adding fuel and providing a rationale for the coming changes was the theory of managed competition. First outlined in the late 1970s by Alain Enthoven, managed competition generally envisioned a strengthening of the demand side—largely in the form of a purchasing cooperative—with individuals (not employers) selecting health insurance plans from among a series of plans offering similar if not identical benefits. Plans would offer a fixed price, as in HMOs, and individuals would pay more when they chose higher-cost plans. Thus managed competition featured some government intervention to level the insurance playing field, greatly enhanced purchasing power in the hands of a sponsor or cooperative, and cost-conscious consumers. The result, it was predicted, would be intense competition between health plans (presumably MCOs), with consumers rewarding those plans that lowered cost, raised quality, or both.

Until the early 1990s, the concept had attracted minimal interest or support. For liberal Democrats it may have leaned too heavily on marketplace competition and was not clearly associated with universal coverage. For Republicans, the concept entailed too much public-sector management, including the establishment of purchasing cooperatives through which employers might be required to purchase insurance and the standardization of health plans and health benefits. In short, for both Democrats and Republicans, managed competition was out of balance. For most Democrats, it relied too heavily on competition; for Republicans, it proposed too much management.

But in the early 1990s, the concept appeared in more varied formulations and drew a sudden growth in interest. An informal group of large employers, insurers, and policy analysts known as the Jackson Hole Group was quietly but effectively spreading the new gospel, at least in the large-employer and insurer communities. Some large employers were beginning to function as miniature purchasing cooperatives, offering employees a choice among competing plans, and making the employees pay more when they chose more expensive plans. The *New York Times* editorial board was waging nothing less than a crusade in support of the concepts. Presidential candidate Paul Tsongas, while offering few details, endorsed it. And in February 1992, two plans—one offered by California Insurance Commissioner John Garamendi,[1] one by the Catholic Health Association—both unequivocally advocating universal coverage, chose managed competition-type con-

---

[1]This plan was based on the deliberations of a commission chaired by the author. The plan was written by the author and staff member Larry Levitt, both of whom—along with several of the commission's members—would later participate in the development and advocacy of the Clinton plan.

structs as the means to the end. In effect, both plans were linking the more conservative, market-oriented features of managed competition with the liberal goal of universal coverage. Thus the proposals offered the compromise of means associated with conservatives to achieve ends associated with liberals. The compromise was duly noted by then–presidential candidate Bill Clinton, among others. Indeed, when the Garamendi plan was first described to Clinton in early 1992, the candidate commented, "It's the best cross I've seen between a competitive marketplace and a single-payer system" (conversation with the author, February 1992).

Most important of all, of course, was the endorsement later that year of managed competition by candidate Clinton, who declared that managed competition, not price controls, would be the driving force in his plan for universal coverage. By October 1992, the *New York Times* editorial board (prematurely) declared the debate to be over; managed competition—still an obscure term understood by only a handful of health care policy wonks—had "won."

All of which, of course, was still nothing but theory. But, especially with Clinton's victory in November, the handwriting was becoming clearer. There was going to be a major effort to enact health care reform, and that effort would promote competition among private health care plans—essentially MCOs—that were likely to be larger, more organized, and under much greater pressure to lower costs.

In early 1993, as the Clinton reform proposal began to take shape, no one doubted that some health care reform was on the horizon. Whatever one's view of the Health Security Act as it emerged, virtually all assumed that the new system would lead to rapid growth in managed care and to more aggressive competition among MCOs. For a while, even the purchasing cooperative, in some form, seemed a likely winner.

By 1994, a minor revolution in health care markets was well under way. Enrollment in MCOs—especially HMOs—began to climb. Hospitals, MCOs, and physicians were consolidating into larger units and exploring new partnerships, largely aimed at securing access to and control over the managed care premium dollar. And health policy and market conferences were focused on the "integrated" or "organized" delivery system, and on the new paradigm in which these systems competed before stronger and more informed purchasers.

By the time health care reform died in the summer of 1994, the genie was out the bottle and gone. Health care reform had lost, and with it went hopes for greater health care security and universal coverage. But marketplace reform, and specifically delivery system reorganization, was proceeding at a pace that was, in many respects at least, faster than any reformer had anticipated.

The Study of Market Change

The study of change at the time of change is never easy. And studying health care market change is no exception to the rule. Much of what passes for information is rumor; much of the remainder is anecdote. There are some good case studies and the beginnings of systemic analysis. But, especially when it comes to assessing the extent of partnering activity (there is better information on the growth of managed care and performance of MCOs), reliable numbers are scarce, and the capacity to assess the impact of developments extremely limited. Figure P.1 breaks out the current status of available information to illustrate the problem.

Not surprisingly, where rumor and anecdote dominate, exaggeration is a likely result. And in reports regarding the changing health care marketplace today, exaggeration is commonplace. For example, there is less direct capitation of individual providers or even of groups of providers than industry and newspaper reports might suggest. There have been fewer actual hospital mergers than anecdotes proclaim, and fewer conversions of hospitals from nonprofit to for-profit status. Purchasing coalitions are growing in number and effectiveness. But aggressive, sophisticated health care purchasing remains very much in the benchmark stage, with few having achieved the ability or leverage of the sponsor envisioned by Enthoven or other managed competition advocates. Declines in premiums trumpeted in national surveys of employers may not, on closer examination, be as significant or as conclusive as first appear to be the case, or as some may want us to believe. The rise of the so-called integrated system is probably—at best—the rise of the *organized* system, with clinical integration proving the hardest form of integration to achieve. And finally, the quality revolution, in

Figure P.1.   Current Status
of Market Analysis by Information Type.

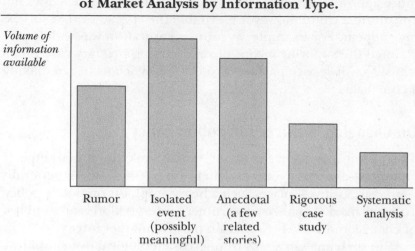

Type of analysis or information

which improved collection and distribution of quality-related information mandates or at least encourages competition on quality, has not yet arrived. It may yet do so. But for the moment, price rules.

Part of the problem is that, as one might expect, those studying market change tend to focus on places where that change is most evident. Current literature on market change is dominated by analysis of developments in California and Minnesota, where HMO penetration is high, where consolidation has been particularly dramatic, and where highly visible and aggressive purchasing organizations (public and private) have had a unique impact on market development. Many assume that California and Minnesota will be bellwether states—that others will follow their leads.

But that may or may not be the case. Both states may prove to be unique, with many features of their delivery systems difficult to emulate. For example, California is marked by the presence of many large medical groups capable of accepting full risk for an insured population. These groups play a critical role in delivery system organization. Other states with few if any such medical groups may find those organizing roles more likely to be filled by hospitals or hospital systems, or by insurers directly, with very different results.

For all these reasons, the concept of benchmarking still seems more appropriate than that of trend. Short-term success does not constitute a trend, however inevitable the spread of that success may appear. For example, as soon as capitation was widely proclaimed the superior means of reimbursing primary care physicians, fee-for-service payments to those physicians began making a comeback.

On Changing Markets and Public Policy

To some, it may seem surprising that a book about marketplace changes—especially one in which those changes are generally viewed as positive—places such a heavy emphasis on public policy. To many market analysts, government intervention is an inhibitor of change and is likely to restrain positive market forces.

But such analysis stems from gross ideological oversimplification. When it comes to health care and health care insurance, in particular, a largely hands-off attitude toward public policy is not a viable option. Not when health care expenditures account for a seventh of the economy. Not when government, still with broad public support, oversees health care programs for the elderly, the poor, and the disabled, and is expected to provide some level of care for others unable to pay. Not when health care costs are the fastest-rising element of government budgets. Not when over forty-three million citizens have no insurance and millions more fear they may lose it. Not when most citizens, given the stakes involved, will expect government to protect them or intervene on their behalf when they believe private enterprises are threatening their interests. And not when market forces, as efficient as they may prove to be, cannot be expected to serve those with no resources with which to purchase marketplace offerings.

And, not, it must be emphasized, when the subject is insurance. Insurance regulation may not always be wisely directed. But insurance always has been and always will be a heavily regulated industry. Two considerations are central here. First, insurance involves a commitment to pay out funds or to deliver services at some point in the future—often a fairly distant future—and insureds need assurance that insurers will be capable of fulfilling the contract. Second, insurers will generally make more profit when they pay out less—in services or dollars. Consumers may have marketplace options when choosing an insurer, but not once they have done so. Thus, there is an almost inherent tension between insureds and insurers, which almost inevitably will lead to consumer demands that government define certain rules by which insurers must abide.

Overall, then, even for those most anxious to allow markets to work, health care policy issues must be addressed. Some government intervention in health care, especially health care insurance markets, is inevitable. Which is not to suggest that policy makers should be rushing to impose their will on marketplace directions. Indeed, one of the wiser policies may be to encourage many flowers to bloom, and to either pursue policies that foster such blooming or reject the efforts of those who might wish to restrain the flowering of some species.

Market-Related Public Policy Options

In a sense, one can define three broad categories of market-related policy options. Most market-focused policy proposals today, and virtually all those to be reviewed or suggested here, would fit into one of the three.

The first category includes efforts to encourage or foster activities that seem fully compatible with market trends, but that might not occur without some policy action. Advocates of such policies, while perhaps admitting that their policies attempt to channel or direct a trend, would argue that those policies are not counter to the trend. In fact, they are likely to be supportive of it, and may even be necessary to clear away impediments to it. For example, moderation of state scope-of-practice laws that restrict various health care professionals (such as, nurse practitioners) from performing certain tasks might be advocated as a means of encouraging integration in delivery systems and of enabling those systems to innovate and lower costs. Enactment of insurance reforms that increase probabilities that insurers will compete on price and quality rather than on ability to avoid high-risk enrollees may be another such policy. Advocates of such reforms would argue that tolerance of insurance industry risk-selection practices will stifle an otherwise positive market trend toward organizational efficiency and productivity driven by competition based on price and quality.

Similar arguments may be offered by those advocating the establishment of small-group purchasing cooperatives, which might enhance the capacity of consumers to choose between competing insurance offerings and thus increase the need of MCOs to improve the value of their products. However, the advocates will assert, such cooperatives may not emerge unless governments give them a push and define some rules that keep them serving the interests of all purchasers.

A second category of policy options entails acceptance of a market trend but recognition of a need to contain or protect against some negative fallout from that trend. For example, one may not wish to interfere with the trend to prepaid health plans or even with the trend to capitation of individual physicians and groups of physicians. At the same time, there may be a need to recognize that under some circumstances strong incentives to reduce utilization can place some groups of individuals at particular risk of underservice. Research suggests, for example, that such groups might include the chronically ill and especially the mentally ill. Thus, even while supporting the capitation trend, policies may be advocated that attempt to establish means by which those most likely to be negatively affected by that trend can be afforded some measure of protection.

On a broader scale, policy makers may recognize that, in a positive vein, current market pressures to secure access to managed care revenue streams and networks can force delivery systems to improve efficiency and lower costs. But it may also be recognized that those same pressures may reduce the willingness of those systems to deliver charity care. Thus some policy options may need to focus on if and how, in this case, the new market-driven system may increase the burden of the public's responsibility to care for the uninsured.

Third, policy choices might include the outright rejection of trends. Policies aimed at restricting market consolidation activity, or at limiting the ability of hospitals to employ physicians or purchase physician practices, or at attempting to expand rate regulation as the primary means of controlling costs would all be examples of such policy. Theoretically, of course, advocates of such policies may object to their proposals being placed in such a category, preferring to view them as modest limitations on otherwise positive trends. Thus, in this policy category many gray areas may emerge. For example, consumer groups may advocate that so-called freedom-of-choice laws, which guarantee rights to seek care outside of networks, are necessary for consumer protection. Others, however, would argue that they restrict the right of MCOs to offer tighter networks (often at lower cost), and therefore are anti-competitive and anti-integration.

Of course, there is always the fourth option. And today, it is often the most popular—do nothing. But in practical terms, doing nothing can be defined as rejecting policies that fall into one of the first three categories. Thus, for example, one may wish to reject so-called any-willing-provider laws, which physician proponents would see as falling into the category of protecting against negative fall-out (loss of physician choice) of managed care. (Opponents, of course, would view such laws as running counter to competition and innovation, and would place them in category three.)

The policy discussions in Chapters Seven through Ten review policy options that at least by the author's definition fall into all three categories. In reviewing them, the primary focus is on the potential advantages and liabilities of policies that might affect the capacity of market forces and trends to achieve public goals—especially, high levels of competition, lower costs and prices, and higher quality. A secondary focus is on policies that may protect consumers and larger public interests from potentially negative impacts of otherwise positive marketplace change.

Analysis Versus Advocacy

Front and center is the question of when and how, if at all, government should intervene. And, as it always has, this will remain a question of continuums, not absolutes. For example, there is probably no business enterprise, big or small, no matter how committed to the "government off the backs of business" philosophy, that has not found the occasion—usually without blinking an ideological eye—to request that a heavier government load be imposed, usually on someone else.

In other words, whatever one's overall philosophical point of view regarding the merits of government intervention, there may always be circumstances in which that philosophy needs to be flexible. This may be particularly so when the playing field is a fast-changing marketplace.

Such is the case with market-oriented health care policy today. Many of the policy issues that arise are new ones, or old ones in new forms or settings. In such circumstances, even analysts with strong ideological convictions or socioeconomic values may find that answers are less than obvious. Perhaps as a result, most of the policy options explored here are more analyzed than advocated.

Part One

The Rise of Managed Care

Chapter One

Making Sense of Trends
The Recent Past and Near Future

When analysts refer to the changing health care marketplace, they may have many trends in mind. But almost any listing of most significant trends would begin with the increasing prominence of managed care, and especially of prepaid HMO plans. This development is marked not just by the increasing numbers of individuals enrolled in managed care plans, but by the increasing acceptance of concepts and strategies—capitation and other forms of risk sharing, reductions in utilization, network selection, and so on—associated with managed care.

However, as managed care continues to grow and prosper—whether defined in terms of numbers of enrollees or strategies deployed—it is not necessarily assuming the forms that many expected it to assume. In fact, a case can be made that in the 1990s managed care, and HMOs in particular, is expanding in large part because it is changing, assuming more flexible and often more consumer-friendly forms, geared to addressing different concerns, in different markets, and at different points in time.

As a result, managed care today assumes many forms, and managed care organizations (MCOs) invoke multiple strategies and appeals: to choice, to quality, to lower price, and so on. In such a fluid environment it is possible to define and discuss trends, but only with the proviso that today's trends are today's trends, and maybe nothing more.

Recent Growth in Managed Care Plans: An Overview

Enrollment in managed care plans, once moderate and consistent, has increased substantially in recent years. And, according to almost all analyses, that rapid growth will continue to expand rapidly in the near future.

The Rise of the HMO

Facilitated by the HMO Act of 1973, which provided start-up grants and loans for HMOs and required large employers to offer HMOs where available, the numbers of individuals in managed care plans rose steadily in the 1980s and even faster in the 1990s. By 1981, HMO enrollment had reached ten million; by 1985, even with the HMO Act no longer in effect, the numbers of HMO enrollees had almost doubled: by 1987, enrollment stood at almost thirty million, and in 1993 at forty-five million. Projections for HMO enrollment by the end of 1995 stood at fifty-six million (Group Health Association of America, 1995a), with estimates of enrollment in 1997 as high as sixty-five million. Figure 1.1 sets out this information in graphic form.

And while the great majority of managed care growth has been in employer-sponsored coverage, by the mid 1990s managed care and especially HMO enrollment is reaching take-off stages in

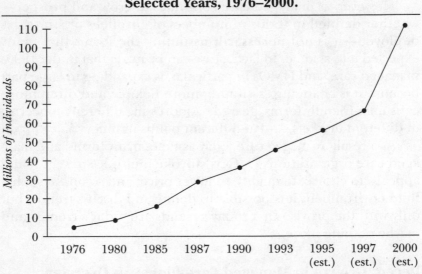

Figure 1.1. Number of Individuals in HMOs: Selected Years, 1976–2000.

Source: Group Health Association of America, 1995a. Estimated figures for 1997 and 2000 come from Hodapp and Samols, 1994.

the publicly funded Medicaid and Medicare programs. Between 1993 and 1994, Medicaid managed care enrollment grew by 69 percent, from 4.8 to 8.1 million beneficiaries (over half of them in HMOs) (Rowland and others, 1994), and is likely to go much higher in the immediate future.

Penetration of HMOs into the Medicare marketplace still lags behind, with less than 10 percent of Medicare's approximately thirty-seven million enrollees in HMOs. Still, Medicare is a fast-growing managed care market. Between 1993 and 1994, the number of Medicare recipients in risk contracts jumped 19 percent and between 1994 and 1995 it increased 27 percent. By January 1995, the number of risk contracts had reached 154, a 41 percent increase in just one year (*Managed Care Outlook*, June 16, 1995).

As enrollment in HMOs rose, so too did enrollment in preferred provider organizations (PPOs), moving from twenty-eight million in 1987 (Shortell and Hull, 1994) to approximately fifty million by the end of 1995. (According to researchers, numbers on PPO enrollment are notoriously poor. This circumstance may reflect a tendency of PPO promoters to inflate their numbers and confusion—especially on the part of those answering research questions—regarding the differences between PPO and point-of-service [POS] plans.) As a result, by the end of 1995, approximately 70 percent of individuals in employer-sponsored plans were in some form of managed care plan. In just seven years, from 1988 to 1995, the traditional fee-for-service insurance plan performed a near-vanishing act, falling from about 70 percent to about 30 percent of the employer-sponsored coverage (Samuelson, 1995; Foster Higgins, 1996). And even the 30 percent was misleading, with most traditional plans now employing at least some managed care usage controls.

Expectations of Greater Future Growth: A National Trend

Looking ahead, all estimates by all sources point to more of the same. While there may be debate about the form the expansion of managed care may take, there is little doubt as to the scope or prospects of continuing change.

Estimates of 10 percent to 15 percent per year growth in HMOs are commonplace, especially if Medicaid and Medicare programs are included in estimates. Such rates of growth would bring

HMO enrollment to over one hundred million by year 2000, a doubling of HMO enrollment in just five years.

A number of factors appear to be responsible for such expectations. Above all, while communities vary widely in extent of managed care or HMO penetration, it is increasingly apparent that the movement to managed care is a national reality, with some of the fastest growth coming, or at least anticipated, in markets (defined by region, community size, and employer size) that for one reason or another have been most resistant. Table 1.1 sets out the growth in terms of percentages enrolled in HMOs by region. From a regional perspective, managed care penetration—especially by HMOs—is increasing everywhere, even in the South, which still lags behind the rest of the nation. Between 1992 and 1995, for example, HMO enrollment (including POS plans) in the Northeast increased from 24 percent of insured workers to 49 percent, while PPO enrollment increased from 8 percent to 17 percent. In the Midwest, PPO enrollment rose by just 1 percent—to 32 percent—but HMO enrollment rose from 21 percent to 35 percent of insured employees (Foster Higgins, 1996).

By market size, while the highest percentages of managed care and HMO enrollees reside in communities of over 1 million, the fastest-growing managed care (a 21 percent increase in HMO enrollees) market is the midsized community of 250,000 to 1 million. And as for size of employer group, a significant movement to

**Table 1.1. Percent Enrolled in HMOs by Region,
1992–1994 (Includes POS Plans).**

	1992 (percent)	*1995 (percent)*	*Growth (percent)*
National	25	41	64
Northeast	24	49	104
South	20	32	60
Midwest	21	35	66
West	36	54	50

Note: Employer-provided insurance only.

Source: 1992 data supplied by Foster Higgins; 1995 data derived from Foster Higgins, 1996.

HMOs is apparent in the midsized employer market, and is even being anticipated in the heretofore most resistant small employer market. Between 1993 and 1995, the penetration of managed care into midsized employee groups grew from 46 to 67 percent (Foster Higgins, 1996). In both 1994 and 1995, the rate of increase in managed care enrollment was greater for employers of less than 500 employees than for those with more than 500 employees (Foster Higgins, 1996).

Among small employers, 1995 HMO penetration remains at a modest 15 percent to 17 percent depending on the definition of small. But it is widely expected to rise—and sharply, largely due to small-group insurance reforms now in place in approximately forty states. These reforms include requirements that all insurers offering products in small-group markets accept any group wishing to purchase that product (known as a *guaranteed issue* provision), and that they base premiums on community rates, or something close to community rates, as opposed to health status or experience of a particular group. Most state laws also limit the imposition of preexisting conditions. In so doing, these reform laws reduce the capacity of traditional indemnity insurers to "cherry pick" the small-group market by offering the lowest-risk groups particularly low rates. Under new state rules, including the movement toward community rating, the playing field between indemnity and HMO plans should level, opening up substantial opportunities for HMOs. According to at least one report, soaring HMO enrollment in New York is, in substantial part, the outgrowth of that state's new community rating law (Hodapp and Samols, 1994). The fact that the small group market has remained a largely untapped HMO market is also, clearly, inspiring increasing competition among HMOs in this market.

Managed Care and Medicaid

Most important, there was the widely held presumption that the Medicaid and Medicare markets were about to become the greatest of managed care growth arenas. In 1995, just one in seven of the approximately seventy million individuals in the two programs was enrolled in a managed care plan, and with state and federal governments desperate to lower their cost, all are looking (perhaps too optimistically) at managed care and HMOs in particular as the answer. Whether the Medicaid program is block-granted to the states or not, states are widely expected to turn to HMOs (with federally approved waivers if necessary) both in hopes of lowering state expenditures, and to unburden themselves of the risk of having to meet rising demands with fewer dollars.

And whereas most HMOs once expressed little interest in Medicaid enrollees, that is hardly the case today. Many HMOs have discovered, reportedly, both that profit can be made in Medicaid managed care and that accepting Medicaid recipients entails much less in the way of administrative, marketing, or other burdens that they may have anticipated. Moreover, they realize that—in an increasingly competitive marketplace—increasing numbers of enrollees (Medicaid enrollees included) increases leverage over providers and appeal for investors.

Perhaps as a result of these and other factors, researchers in the Robert Wood Johnson Foundation-sponsored "Health System Change" project reported in December 1995 that in several markets the entry of new plans was significant, and largely attributable to expectations of increases in Medicaid managed care enrollment. Anecdotal reports from other markets confirm that competition for Medicaid enrollees in several states has become intense, with plans willing to accept Medicaid enrollments at prices once deemed inconceivable. Figure 1.2 gives a graphic picture of the trend.

Managed Care and Medicare

On the Medicare front, the situation is more complicated. For one thing, resistance to HMOs among many seniors remains high. In 1995, Congressional Republicans had to abandon a managed competition-type plan in which recipients would be provided a fixed dollar benefit rather than a fixed package of services. Such a plan (or even an alternative in which Medicare would pay for the low-cost plan only) would almost certainly force seniors choosing the traditional fee-for-service Medicare system to pay significantly more than if they were to enroll in an HMO.

Additionally, federal regulators at the Health Care Financing Administration (HCFA) continue to struggle with Medicare risk adjustment issues. Under current arrangements, HCFA reports, it loses money when seniors enroll in HMOs, which, it reports, attract

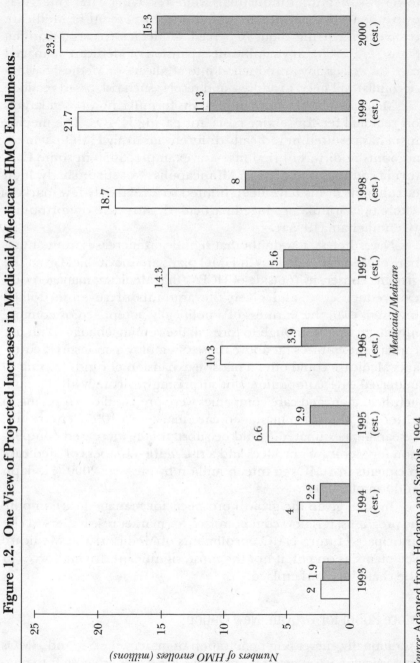

Figure 1.2. One View of Projected Increases in Medicaid/Medicare HMO Enrollments.

Source: Adapted from Hodapp and Samols. 1994.

lower-risk, healthier individuals while receiving what emerge as overly generous payments. With about 10 percent of Medicare recipients incurring about 70 percent of Medicare costs ("Warning Signs . . . ," 1995), any significant expansion of Medicare managed care (as well as any introduction into Medicare of Medical Savings Accounts) will need to address and resolve such risk-based realities.

Medicare also needs to improve its formula, now based largely on regional fee-for-service costs, for paying HMOs. The mechanism has resulted in radically different monthly HMO payment amounts in different regions—for example, $650 in some California counties and $350 in Minneapolis. Not surprisingly, high enrollment levels have been limited to a relatively few markets where the formula produced particularly attractive opportunities (Cunningham, 1995a).

Nevertheless, few doubt that significant increases in the numbers of Medicare eligibles in HMO plans are inevitable. Given the growing consensus (outside of HCFA) that Medicare managed care can reduce costs and given the amounts of revenue dollars involved, even the wariness of a politically potent senior community might not be enough to forestall the coming change. With per capita expenditures far above those of employer-sponsored coverage, Medicare could offer a massive expansion of funds flowing to managed care companies. Not surprisingly, virtually all the publicly held managed care companies were prepared or preparing to enter the Medicare managed care market in 1995. The result, researchers estimated, could be substantially increased competition for Medicare enrollees and a rise in the numbers of Medicare recipients in HMOs to fifteen million by the year 2000 (Hodapp and Samols, 1994).

In sum, given the growth prospects for managed care in public programs, it is now commonplace for market researchers to cite anticipated future HMO enrollments of Medicaid and Medicare recipients as one of, if not the most, significant driving forces in the changing marketplace.

More Room for Growth: New Options

Additionally, increasing penetration of managed care, and HMOs in particular, is expected because there is still so much left to penetrate. In spite of all the dramatic growth, less than 20 percent of the U.S. population was in HMOs in 1995. Three-quarters of the nation's 258 metropolitan markets had less than 25 percent of their populations in HMOs ("Mid-Sized Firms Embrace MCOs," 1995). Clearly, so long as managed care plans can offer employers (self-insured included) lower premiums than traditional plans, as is increasingly the case today, the proverbial handwriting would seem to be on the wall, at least with regard to traditional plans. As to the movement from PPOs to HMOs, the issue is more complicated. The latter, clearly, offer lower overall costs, but because more of the cost of PPOs is borne by the employees in cost-sharing, premiums paid by employers are still usually less than those paid for HMOs.

Finally, ongoing growth in managed care enrollment, especially HMO enrollment, is widely anticipated because HMOs may finally have discovered the means (indeed, some wonder why it took so long) of surmounting one of the industry's greatest hurdles: the perception, and reality, that HMOs deny choice of physician. The POS option, offering the HMO enrollee an option to go out of net-work (albeit at higher cost), and, to a lesser extent, the independent practice association (IPA) model HMO (often offering greater numbers of physician members, and thus more choice) appear to have struck positive chords with those who may be looking for a compromise between HMO price and fee-for-service choice.

The Staying Power of Choice: IPAs, PPOs, and POS Plans

Before undertaking an analysis of which forms of managed care may be experiencing the greatest growth, one point must be emphasized: The terminology used to describe different types of HMOs is far behind the times, and may be close to losing all relevance. IPA models, for example, generally defined as (predominantly loose) associations of independent physicians that contract with an HMO, often include many physicians in group practices, and may even be organized by or built around a group practice. And the arrangement in which an HMO contracts with several different multispecialty groups, with each serving a defined population of HMO patients, might be defined (depending upon definitions and perspective employed) as a *network* model (the HMO is contracting with many medical groups); a *group* model (all enrollees in a particular plan are going, exclusively, to a particular medical group); or an *IPA/network* model, where a medical group employs its affiliated IPA to deliver care.

The terminology breakdown results from several factors, including a fundamental confusion over whether the *type* of HMO refers to the MCO (for example PacifiCare or Prudential) or to the structure of the particular plan or plans it may be offering. But the breakdown seems to be related primarily to the reality that most MCOs are offering several different models in different regions, and even sometimes in the same region; and the plans being offered are, increasingly, hybrid networks featuring all kinds of combinations of large groups, small groups, and independent practitioners, most of whom have contracts with a number of MCOs. The result of these two trends can be depicted as the movement of increasing numbers of HMO arrangements into box D on Table 1.2.

For researchers hoping to compare HMO forms—according to performance, physician payment mechanisms, exclusive or nonexclusive contractual relationships, or countless other variables—the situation is close to hopeless, especially where the goal is to compare systems over time, during which they are likely to change.

And most important, from a market-study perspective, is the reality that the categories or plan types, such as they are, are of almost no value in describing HMO arrangements to consumers. With the possible exception of the traditionally defined staff or group models, in which the consumer goes to one clearly definable organization of physicians often practicing in one place, all the models and hybrids may look the same; the consumer can go to some

Table 1.2. Classifying HMOs by Nature of Plans Offered.

	Pure	*Hybrid*
HMO offers one type of HMO plan (for example, staff model)	A	B
HMO offers multiple plans (for example, group and IPA)	C	D

groups or individual physicians and not others—unless they pay an additional or higher charge. Indeed, where HMO co-payments rise significantly beyond the $5 to $10 charge, even the differences (again, from the consumer's point of view) between PPOs and HMOs can begin to break down. The growth of POS plans, of course, renders this breakdown all the more likely, as differences between these plans and PPOs often become indistinguishable.

The Rise of the IPA

Whatever the definition, though, managed care—and HMO enrollment in particular—has soared. But not due to the rise of the highly integrated, one-stop, limited-choice HMO model that many, until fairly recently, thought would dominate the industry. In fact, the dramatic growth in managed care and HMOs has occurred largely because managed care has changed, perhaps adapting to continuing consumer and employer requirements of choice. Today, nearly three-quarters of all managed care enrollees are in a plan with a choice option; and nearly all the increase in managed care enrollment between 1993 and 1994 came in plans with an out-of-network option (Cunningham, 1995b).

Thus, while enrollment in group and staff model HMOs has remained flat (at least in terms of percentages of enrollees), enrollment in generally less integrated network or IPA-type models, especially those with a POS option, is rising rapidly. Between 1989 and 1994, the percentage of HMO enrollees in network and IPA models (if these terms may still be employed) rose from 58 to 69 percent, while the percentage of enrollees in group and staff models fell from 42 to 31 percent. (See Table 1.3.) Nearly two-thirds (8.1 million individuals) of total HMO growth between the end of 1992 and the end of 1994 was in IPA plans (data calculated from Group Health Association of America, 1995a).

There would appear to be a host of explanations for why MCOs, providers, and even consumers have moved toward the IPA model, or at least toward HMO plans employing generally broad networks of physicians and groups. From the MCO's viewpoint, the first reality is often one of the absence of options. In many parts of the country, there are few (if any) large group practices around which a group or staff model might be built. IPAs are also

Table 1.3. Percent of HMO Enrollees by Type of Plan.

Type of Plan	End, 1989	End, 1994
Staff	12	11
Group	30	20
Network	15	19
IPA	43	50

Source: Based on data from Group Health Association of America, 1995a.

far simpler and less expensive to organize, entailing little of the investment in bricks and mortar or long-term contracts that generally accompany the organization of more integrated models. As such, they may be more flexible and easier to expand (or contract) as necessary, and appear to be particularly appropriate when the task is new and fast market entry.

IPA/network approaches may also meet the requirements of many physicians. While recognizing the need to venture into managed care arrangements, many may still hope to maintain some vestige of independent practice, including the opportunity to contract with a variety of MCOs. The fact that contractual arrangements are often made with a physician-led organization (which in turn contracts with an HMO) may also have appeal to participating physicians.

As for consumers, IPA/network-type models may offer the appearance—and if they are large enough the reality—of more choice. This, of course, will be especially true if they offer a POS option, as increasing numbers do.

In the marketplace, however, it is not the innate appeal of a model that may determine its success; it is its ability to perform. In today's market, above all, that may mean the ability to compete on price, and judged by that yardstick there remains considerable debate concerning the staying power of the IPA approach.

Skeptics point to analyses offered by some researchers, including the Congressional Budget Office (CBO), that IPAs have shown little capacity to reduce utilization. While the CBO has significantly raised its estimate of reduced utilization in staff and group models, its research review continues to conclude that IPAs have produced only minimal decreases in utilization (Christensen, 1995). In addition, as the CBO emphasizes, any-willing-provider laws (if approved in states) and POS options could be potentially very damaging to the ability of IPAs to reduce utilization. Any-willing-provider laws would have similar effects on staff and group models, but these are more likely to be exempted from the law's provisions. Thus, not only do any-willing-provider laws limit the IPA's capacity to control utilization, they also may harm the IPA's competitive posture as well.

As for POS options, they may appeal to high-cost enrollees, more attracted to the security offered by opt-out provisions. As a result, IPAs offering POS plans (as they are more and more likely to do) could suffer from adverse selection—both in terms of who they enroll and in how often their enrollees go out of network.

Finally, as more organized delivery systems (ODSs) emerge, featuring improved communications systems, greater capacity to implement protocols, higher levels of physician-system integration and stronger management styles, the IPA/network approach may be relegated to an untenable competitive position. The new systems may be more capable of lowering costs, improving quality, and demonstrating higher quality. And, just as important, as physicians acknowledge the new paradigm of the organized system, those systems may become more acceptable to physicians and thus more appealing than independent network arrangements.

On the other hand, assessments of IPAs and their potential to reduce costs—such as those conducted by the CBO—may focus on aggregate numbers when benchmarks are far more revealing and perhaps more relevant. Most IPAs may remain loose, minimally integrated organizations of independent practitioners. But, in California especially, a wholly different breed of IPAs seems to be emerging. These organizations are strengthening governance structures, invoking more aggressive management styles (including more extensive and more sophisticated profiling of providers), increasing financial and other ties between physicians and the organization, and employing aggressive capitation strategies—focused on the individual physician or group of physicians—to reduce utilization of hospitals and specialists.

According to some researchers and to data provided by organizations representing these IPAs, many California IPAs are approaching the standards achieved by the best of group HMO models on critical indicators of utilization such as hospital days per thousand. The best-performing California IPAs have reportedly reduced hospitalization rates by 40 percent and specialty utilization by 60 percent, and have lowered commercial hospital days per thousand enrollees to under 200 (Governance Committee, 1995, pp. 83, 90), as compared to national HMO averages of 270 (Gabel and others, 1994, p. 23) and a California HMO average of 229 (Governance Committee, 1994, p. 20).

In effect, then, the IPA debate may be one of definition. IPAs as they came to be known—as loose affiliations of independent physicians—may have little staying power, at least in mature managed care markets. But the newer California-type IPAs function more like medical groups and group model HMOs. In fact, some have been organized by large California medical groups (such as the Mullikin Group) in a kind of wrap-around package, with the medical group often using some of its IPA physicians to service portions of the group's managed care contracts.

The overall result can be an IPA of independent physicians and practices that is a virtual medical group. Its physicians maintain their formal independence, but in terms of organization, communication, utilization strategies, and so on, the IPA can be very much a group. As such a relationship, the new IPA, or network of independent physicians, may be defining a more viable balance between physician autonomy and physician accountability.

POS Plans: New Forms and New Growth

Accompanying—and in many respects fueling—the rise of the IPA is the sudden expansion of the POS plan. Under this option, individuals enroll in HMOs, but have the option to seek care outside the network, usually with higher cost sharing in both deductibles and co-payments. While care through network providers may entail no deductibles and no co-payments, going out of the network may invoke a deductible of perhaps $250, and cost-sharing of 20 percent to 30 percent. Thus, POS plans are often referred to as *hybrids,* being part HMO—a fixed, prepayment—and part indemnity plan—a percentage-of-provider-charge payment when using out-of-plan providers.

According to anecdotal reports, POS options are sweeping the nation. It is difficult to get a firm reading on just how "sweeping" the trend may be because of the hybrid nature of POS plans. Estimates of numbers of enrollees in POS plans vary widely, even among diligent researchers. Additionally, some view all POS plans as HMOs, whereas others view only some as HMOs. Indeed, if all POS plans were viewed as HMOs—as perhaps should be the case—the numbers of individuals in HMOs as of 1995 might be closer to 60 or 65 million enrollees than to the 56 million enrollees generally cited. But whatever the definition employed, the numbers of POS plans and enrollment in them have risen substantially.

- Between 1992 and 1994, the percentage of insured employees in POS plans rose from 4 percent to 15 percent.
- Between 1990 and 1993, the percentage of HMOs offering a POS option grew from under 20 percent to almost 60 percent (Gabel, 1994).
- The number of large employers offering POS plans increased from 15 percent in 1993 to 28 percent in 1995 (Foster Higgins, 1996).
- By mid-1995, POS plans may have had, depending on different estimates and definitions, somewhere around twenty million enrollees.

By mid 1995, even Kaiser Permanente, the organization most synonymous with the concept of restricted networks, was moving to include out-of-network options. As part of larger efforts to adjust to changing market circumstances, Kaiser introduced preferred provider organization (PPO) products in Kansas City and California markets, and was introducing POS products in a number of markets ("Sick People in Managed Care . . . ," 1995).

Still, the question remains, as it does with PPO and IPA trends: are POS option plans likely to remain as a semipermanent fixture in the managed care marketplace? Or, are they more likely to emerge as a transitional phase, a step toward more traditional and more limited HMO choice models?

Point of Service: A Skeptical View

Skeptics can make a good case. As might be expected, POS is more expensive than other HMO forms, by perhaps as much as 20 percent (Palzbo and others, 1993), and 1994 employer premium increases were higher in POS plans (about 10 percent as opposed to 6.4 percent for non-POS HMOs and 2.1 percent for PPOs (Service, 1995). In 1995, premiums for POS plans rose by 3.4 percent, and premiums for other HMOs fell by 3.8 percent, a differential of over 7 percent (Foster Higgins, 1996). Over a few years, such a trend could soon price the POS option out of business.

Such will be the case, almost certainly, if the higher costs reflect fundamental flaws in the construct. If the POS option encourages significant out-of-network utilization, the capacity of an HMO to lower cost and to coordinate care across providers could be critically undermined. The utility, for example, of cost-effective protocols could be greatly diminished if patients availed themselves of other options—for example to see out-of-network specialists—when protocols might have the greatest value.

Additionally, POS plans, as noted above, may be prone to two forms of negative pricing spiral. First, efforts to keep the option attractive by holding down patient cost-sharing could increase out-of-network utilization, perhaps increasing system costs and compounding coordination-of-care concerns. Second, POS option plans may also suffer from adverse selection, attracting less healthy, higher-cost individuals, who may be particularly interested in maintaining and utilizing out-of-network options.

Point of Service Staying Power

In spite of these liabilities, however, most observers believe the POS option has considerable potential for growth. Indeed, some believe that the growth of POS and other hybrid, choice-oriented managed care plans have produced a step-level change in public acceptance of managed care, offering greater assurances of choice and quality (defined by many as choice) than can be found in more restricted HMO settings (Meyer and others, 1994).

Most important, perhaps, are findings suggesting that, to date at least, use of the POS option by those in plans offering it has been modest. Only about 16 percent of enrollees use the out-of-network option (Gabel and others, 1994), and there is reason to anticipate that such levels might decline. A *New York Times* survey, for example, found that the utilization of out-of-network services declines as HMOs get larger and more mature, and as enrollees, many of whom come to POS HMO plans from fee-for-service plans, stay in them longer. The *Times* review also suggested that out-of-network usage may be lower where managed care penetration is higher and managed care more accepted. For example, in Minnesota, where HMO penetration is high, some plans reported out-of-network spending of as low as 4 percent (Freudenheim, 1995d). Such findings suggest that as POS options are offered to enrollees accustomed to managed care and its restrictions—as opposed to enrollees coming in from traditional insurance relationships—out-of-network utilization should decline.

Under these circumstances, premiums for POS plans may come down. Indeed, some suggest that their present elevated levels may reflect, in part, HMO uncertainty regarding out-of-network utilization. Premiums could also be reduced if deductibles or co-payments on out-of-network services were increased. But even assuming higher premiums for the POS option, consumers may feel the extra perceived protection well worth it.

PPOs

The outlook for PPOs is less clear. Even as many PPOs have become more aggressive in invoking managed care strategies, many analysts believe that their future, or at least their capacity to grow, is limited. Their structure, still linked to indemnity insurance and discounted fee-for-service payments, seems unlikely to reduce utilization and costs far enough to effectively compete on overall cost with more aggressively managed and more integrated managed care models.

For these reasons, many believe that current PPO resilience and growth result largely from their service as a transition phase through which individuals move from fee-for-service to HMO plans. For example, enrollment numbers from the South seem to support this analysis. In that region, the percent of employees in PPOs rose substantially, from 30 percent to 39 percent, between 1994 and 1995. By contrast, the percent of employees enrolled in traditional fee-for-service plans fell from 42 percent to 29 percent (Foster Higgins, 1996). Such a theory of transition may also be relevant for self-insured plans. In these plans, PPOs are particularly common, partly because employees may resist HMOs and partly because HMOs are generally insured products, and purchasing them gives up advantages employers see in self-insurance.

Indications of a potential decline of the PPO may also be found in slowing rates of growth in PPO enrollment. Although the numbers of PPOs have continued to grow (from 681 in 1992 to 802 in 1994), the rate of increase in PPO enrollment—according to at least one report—has fallen from 56 percent in 1992, to 32 percent in 1993, to just 3.2 percent in 1994 (Fubini and Antonelli, 1996).

For now, however, predictions of the demise of the PPO seem clearly premature. In some respects, PPOs are still showing substantial growth, with the percent of HMOs offering PPO products almost doubling between 1990 and 1993 (Gabel and others, 1994), and the percent of insured employees in PPO plans remaining constant, in the high twenties, over the past few years. Today, as noted earlier, approximately 50 million individuals are enrolled in PPOs.

Moreover, beyond the numbers, the logic of PPOs remains valid. Above all, because much of their cost is paid by the enrollee in cost-sharing, premiums remain low. Today, according to at least one survey, PPO premiums nationwide are below—albeit just below—those of HMOs (Foster Higgins, 1996). Thus, although the PPO arrangement will almost always cost the employee more, due to higher cost-sharing and less extensive benefits, it may cost the employer less, and it is the latter who is usually choosing the plan.

Moreover, especially when contrasted with the restrictions generally associated with HMOs, PPOs continue to offer the image—and sometimes the reality—of more consumer choice. Indeed, for consumers demanding significant choice options, PPOs may still maintain advantages over POS HMO plans. Especially if deductibles and co-payments in the PPO remain modest, these two options will look much the same from the consumer's point of view, whatever distinctions policy analysts may draw between discounted fee-for-service and risk-sharing plans. And from the consumer's point of view, the PPO may maintain its association with choice and fee-for-service, while the POS option, although also offering choice, includes an association with an HMO.

Additionally, PPOs may remain a preferred organizational mode of many emerging physician networks. And so long as excess capacity—especially of specialists and hospitals—remains as high as it does today, PPOs may find that high levels of physician insecurity render the available discounts in discounted fee-for-service very deep, getting them a long way toward lower costs.

Finally, the PPO approach can be linked to the most integrated of delivery systems. Today, many HMOs and many ODSs—in addition to contracting with or operating their own HMOs—will rent out their provider network to insurers and self-insured employers operating PPO plans. In this way, PPOs can benefit from the increased coordination and efficiency associated with more integrated managed care systems while still offering a valued choice option to consumers.

Trends in Premiums and Costs

Trends are down—but what do they mean?

Figures released in early 1995 trumpeted another year of declining health insurance costs. The surveys suggested that rates of premium increase for HMOs in particular were continuing on a downward trend, from double digits just a few years ago (15 percent in 1990), to ranges of 6 percent and less in 1994 and 1995 (Service, 1995; "Health Benefits in 1994," 1995).

Heralded with even greater fanfare was the finding that for the first time in two decades, employers of over ten individuals experienced an actual reduction (1.1 percent) in overall per employee health care costs (Service, 1995).

Employer surveys of premiums in 1995 reflected similar trends. Although figures indicated a slight rise in overall employer per employee costs, the rise appeared to be almost totally attributable to rising costs of traditional indemnity plans and especially to rising numbers of retirees in those plans. For active employees HMO premiums fell by almost 4 percent from 1994 levels. According to one research organization at least, this was the first time in ten years of survey activity that employee HMO premiums actually declined (Foster Higgins, 1996). PPO costs also declined—by 2.1 percent.

And, just as significant, the decline in costs appeared to be reaching smaller (less than 500 employees) as well as larger employers. As many survey and anecdotal reports suggest, managed care penetration in small- and mid-employer markets is increasing, and with that increase is coming more intense competition. Lower premiums is one likely result.

As discussed below, employer surveys have significant limitations; most specifically, falling premiums or employer costs do not necessarily reflect lower overall health care costs. But the accumulation of evidence did appear to indicate that MCOs were holding premium increases down, and that the gap between managed care and indemnity plan premiums was widening—which over time would spell rising enrollment for managed care plans.

For employers (especially those taking leadership in the new demand-side efforts), for the managed care industry (promoting greater performance and cost reductions without government intervention), and for the promoters of integrated systems and the consultants they hired, these were heady results. The case for the superiority of managed care—HMOs and integrated systems in particular—in controlling skyrocketing health care costs appeared stronger than ever.

As outlined in the Prologue, from a broad marketplace perspective the explanation for reduced premiums lay not just in the rise of managed care, but in the continuing shift from competition between fee-for-service and managed care to competition among managed care options. As market penetration of managed care rises, shadow pricing of fee-for-service plans gives way to pressure to reduce utilization and costs, thus enabling premiums to decline and market share, it is hoped, to rise.

And although, as will be discussed shortly, many remain skeptical regarding the long-term prospects of managed care to reduce utilization and costs, it is getting harder to deny a certain logic in the case for managed care, especially if the focus is on key regions and benchmark plans rather than on the nation as a whole. In HMOs, particularly in staff and group models but even in some IPAs, hospital utilization rates—computed in hospital days per thousand enrollees, average lengths of stay, or admission rates—were well below those of traditional insurance plans. And, at least in many regions, they were continuing to fall. By 1992, for example, the average days per thousand (for those under sixty-five) was at about 456 for all insurance plans (including HMOs) but 270 for HMOs alone. For the over sixty-five population (Medicare enrollees, essentially), the comparable figures were 2,772 and 1,295, respectively. For West Coast plans, where managed care penetration was higher and competition between managed care plans greater, the numbers were significantly lower (Gabel and others, 1994). By 1995, some HMOs and large capitated medical groups were reporting hospital days per thousand in California for the under sixty-five population as 170 or less and for the over sixty-five population at 960 or less (Hodapp and Samols, 1994; Robinson and Casalino, 1995). (Different sources employ different methodologies in calculating such measures as hospital days per thousand, so figures from different studies may not be fully comparable. However, there isn't much question that the trend has been down, and particularly so in California.) Some are estimating that, with some increased utilization of home care, hospital days per thousand for the under sixty-five enrollees could soon fall to below 140. See Figure 1.3 for a depiction of hospital utilization.

There is also increasing evidence, from many studies, that HMOs reduce the utilization of specialists and of high-cost tests and procedures (Shortell and Hull, 1994) and are achieving significant shifts from inpatient to outpatient settings. To be sure, data from Medicare and Medicaid were more mixed and somewhat less compelling. One review concluded, for example, that HMOs had not lowered inpatient utilization in the Medicaid program (Shortell and Hull, 1994), nor had they lowered admissions in the Medicare program. Even so, the same review revealed that HMOs had reduced average lengths of stay for Medicare enrollees, and evidence from Arizona's statewide alternative Medicaid program featuring mandatory enrollment in managed care plans lowered costs compared to traditional Medicaid programs by 19 percent per enrollee. Additionally, as suggested by increasing competition among HMOs for Medicaid enrollees in many states, many HMOs at least anticipate providing Medicaid benefits at lower costs.

There was even some evidence that the old assumption that HMOs attracted healthier enrollees (thus facilitating more significant cost reductions) might no longer be valid, at least with regard to the chronically ill. A study published in early 1995 found little difference in the prevalence of 15 chronic conditions among those enrolled in HMO or indemnity plans ("Do HMOs Care . . . ," 1995).

Support for the proposition that managed care can continue to reduce costs also comes from the levels of excess capacity in the system, and from the leverage that excess offers MCOs in bargaining with providers. Hospitals nationwide are operating at less than

Figure 1.3. Differences in Hospital Utilization in 1992.

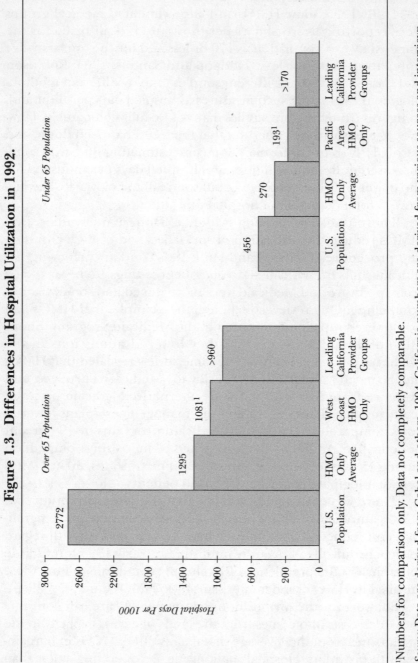

Over 65 Population

Under 65 Population

Hospital Days Per 1000

U.S. Population	2772	
HMO Only Average	1295	
West Coast HMO Only	1081[1]	
Leading California Provider Groups	>960	
U.S. Population	456	
HMO Only Average	270	
Pacific Area HMO Only	193[1]	
Leading California Provider Groups	>170	

[1]Numbers for comparison only. Data not completely comparable.

Source: Data are derived from Gabel and others, 1994. California numbers are derived from various sources and interviews.

two-thirds of capacity. Many specialties are overpopulated (based on HMO needs) by factors of 100 percent to 200 percent or more. Even the vaunted shortage of primary care physicians is disappearing, with some markets already approaching surplus and adequate supplies of primary care physicians, nationwide, expected by year 2000 (Epstein, 1995a).

In the days of indemnity insurance, when supply ruled demand, and when costs were just passed from physicians to insurer to employers, who paid continually higher premiums, such excess capacity tended to raise rather than lower costs. Studies found that excess capacity in a region led not to lower prices—as economists would generally anticipate—but to greater volume of services. But in the era of competing MCOs and more aggressive buyers, the demand side reasserts itself. Physicians, especially specialists, find their services in less demand, and MCOs, pressured in turn by employers, demand lower prices.

The logic of such numbers is clear. Today, most health care markets are increasingly buyer's markets, and will be for some time. In increasing numbers of markets, it seems likely that MCOs will be paying for fewer units of utilization, and also paying less for each unit.

To this systematically collected evidence can be added analysis of a more anecdotal nature suggesting that in many markets managed care has just begun to produce savings, and that even in mature markets, additional savings are still being generated. Many believe that direct capitation of physicians and physician groups can reduce utilization and costs, and there is some systematically collected data to support this view (Miller and Luft, 1993). Yet, as we shall see in Chapter Two, the great majority of physicians and medical groups are still being reimbursed by traditional discounted fee-for-service measures. Capitation of hospitals remains rare. There is, in other words, a great deal of room for expansion of the capitation strategy.

Additionally, utilization of hospital and other services varies widely from state to state, suggesting substantial room for improvement in many regions. For example, average length of stay for Medicare enrollees in Los Angeles was 8.2 days in 1992; in New York City, it was 13.2 (Hodapp and Samols, 1994). In California, commercial days per thousand enrollees averaged 229 days in

HMOs (and 133 days in so-called best practice HMOs) in 1993. Comparable average figures were 330 for Georgia, and 335 for New York (Governance Committee, 1994); the national HMO average (for 1992) stood at about 270 (Palzbo and others, 1993).

In short, in most markets—including mature markets—there is considerable evidence that utilization can be further reduced. Thus, in the words of many practitioners and researchers, "We don't really know where the bottom is."

Similar to wide differences in utilization are wide differences in premiums across states. Whatever their limitations as a measuring stick (and they are significant), these differences were often 25 percent or more—even between HMOs. While premiums in 1995 in California were estimated at around $115 per month for individuals in employer-sponsored plans, premiums for comparable benefits packages in Massachusetts, where HMO penetration was also high, were in the $140–$150 range. These differences may reflect many factors beyond underlying costs, but it appears likely that at least some of the differences are attributable to lower costs driven by more efficient delivery systems.

To all of which, finally, could be added the reality that both competition between MCOs and increasing pressure from employers for lower costs are still fairly modern phenomena. As noted earlier, three-quarters of the nation's 258 metropolitan markets had HMO penetration rates of less than 25 percent in 1995. And, in spite of attention and praise gathered by a few large employer-purchasing groups, employers were only just beginning to form the kinds of purchasing coalitions that might maximize the power of the purchaser.

Such is the body of evidence, systematic and anecdotal, that MCOs—especially HMOs—can reduce both costs and premiums relative to traditional insurance plans, and that they can continue to do so over time. Even if incomplete, that evidence is substantial, especially if we focus on market leaders—regions or plans—rather than national averages.

Premiums and Costs: A Few Significant Caveats

Some health policy analysts and economists, however, remain skeptical, and with some justification. Most significantly, they note that

Is California the Future?

The Advisory Board, a private research agency, has compiled the following numbers on the California marketplace. Much of the information, clearly, is anecdotal, based on interviews with and data collected from individual MCOs and delivery systems.

- California premiums are falling; they are now at about $110 per member per month.
- California's most organized and aggressive purchasers, the California Public Employees Retirement System (CalPERS) and the Pacific Business Group on Health, have seen overall premiums decline by upwards of 5 percent in 1995.
- California capitation rates are below those seen in other regions. In California, full professional capitation rates (primary and specialty care) are running $35–$40. Comparable numbers in other cities are: Houston, $45–$50; Chicago, $41–$46; New York, $59; Atlanta, $45.
- In Southern California, some specialty capitation rates have fallen as much as 33 percent between 1994 and 1995.
- Much of the reduction in California premiums is being fueled by falling physician incomes. Physician pretax income in California rose by an average annual increase of 7 percent between 1991 and 1994, peaking at $161,000 in 1994. Estimated physician income for 1995 is $144,000; for 1996, $122,000; and for 1997, $101,000; overall, an average annual decrease of 15 percent (Governance Committee, 1995).

premiums for HMOs (with the exception of the most recent data on 1995) are still rising—often at rates two or three times that of inflation. The reduction in employer costs, it is important to acknowledge, has generally resulted not from falling premiums, but from one-time shifts from traditional insurance plans to lower-cost managed care plans.

Moreover, reductions in premium levels can result from many short-term forces—reductions in benefits, increased utilization of specialty carve-outs (for high-cost services) or price wars—that have little to do with underlying costs. It is widely reported, for example, that in some of the most competitive managed care markets, many MCOs are pricing below cost and losing money in the battle for market share. In such cases, what may appear to be lower costs may in fact be lower profits, certainly a time-bound circumstance.

Clearly, short-term or one-time factors that might be responsible for reducing premiums do not demonstrate a long-term, ongoing capacity to reduce underlying costs—that is, costs associated with something more than one-time savings.

HMOs, skeptics may acknowledge, are less expensive, perhaps 5 percent to 15 percent less expensive than traditional plans, depending upon the region. (And that difference, it should be noted, does not usually include the additional benefits and cost-sharing HMOs offer.) But research has not yet conclusively demonstrated that HMOs can produce ongoing—that is, more than one-time—savings.

In addition to these fundamental issues of capacity to generate more than one-time savings, a number of other factors suggest that predictions of ongoing reductions in premiums or rates in growth thereof may be premature.

Above all, medical capabilities continue to expand, increasing the ability of medicine to perform more services, often at higher costs. And although some technological advances (for example, a drug therapy that substitutes for a surgical procedure) can lower costs, most analysts conclude that improved capabilities (including technological advances) are more likely to raise costs. Generally, this is because the new technology or treatment is more expensive than the old one (for example, MRIs compared to X-rays), or because the new technology, even if inexpensive, enables providers to bring comfort and better health to far greater numbers of patients, thus resulting in more medical interventions and higher utilization of medical services.

To the matter of increasing capability must be added the aging factor and the nation's apparent unwillingness to address ethical issues of when doing more is appropriate—that is, the rationing issue. These factors may produce (especially once the most obvious instances of overutilization are reduced) as much upward pressure on utilization, costs, and premiums as improving managed care techniques are likely to produce in downward pressure. All of which, of course, is not a criticism of managed care. The point is that whatever the capacity of managed care to lower costs, other factors pushing costs upward may have as great or greater force.

Public demands for choice may also limit the capacity of managed care to reduce costs and premiums. As we have seen, plans offering more choice tend to be more expensive. Even more significant, they are the fastest growing of managed care plans. Yet, for the most part, the HMO systems with the greatest proven track record of lower utilization tend to be the staff and group models that are more restrictive of choice. Their growth rate has been flat.

There may also be limits to the ability of MCOs to reduce costs and premiums by leveraging providers whose bargaining positions are undermined by the existence of excess capacity. As we shall soon see, providers are reorganizing and consolidating, in large part to defend current revenue levels. And while excess capacity is considerable in many markets, it can be expected to decline over time. As it does, the bargaining hand of providers will be strengthened.

Increased competition, too, for all its trumpeted values, may exact a price. As markets move from those in which rising costs were just passed along to those in which major MCOs compete more aggressively, marketing costs may rise—and dramatically. This should prove true not just for MCOs, but for delivery systems that will find it necessary to persuade employers and consumers that no network is complete without them. "Do not join any HMO without making sure you can come to us!" is already becoming a common radio refrain.

Lastly, there is the issue of smaller employers, the individual market, and the question of systemwide costs. Large and even mid-sized employers may be paying less for insurance, but others may be seeing fewer benefits of the new revolution.

As surveys make clear, the greatest gains in premium reductions have been experienced by the largest employers. Small employers, even though they are shifting more employees to managed care plans, are still experiencing per person premium increases (over 6 percent in 1994) of at least twice current inflation levels (Service, 1995).

And, most significantly, the number of individuals insured in the individual market (where premiums are generally well above group rates) and the number of uninsured individuals are both growing substantially, due in large part to decreases in the number of employers covering workers, and increases in contractual arrangements between employers and workers, self-employed individuals, and part-time workers. In just one year, from 1993 to 1994, the individual market grew by 2.3 million ("The Number of Americans . . . ," 1995). And by the end of 1995, the uninsured numbered 43 million, and were likely to be in the neighborhood of 50 million by the turn of the century. These populations—those insured as individuals and those without insurance, including the unemployed and many of the nation's most vulnerable populations—have always included relatively high proportions of the highest-cost individuals.

Thus, all told, there must remain some concern that at least some of the lower costs and premiums now benefiting those with the strongest purchasing power may be resulting in some cost shifting onto smaller employers and the individual and uninsured marketplaces. It is this kind of logic that leads health economists to uncertainty on the issue of whether lower costs and premiums seen in managed care plans today are actually reducing system costs overall.

If a conclusion must be reached, then, it is that both the advocates of managed care and the skeptics may be right. Managed care does seem capable of reducing utilization and costs, and perhaps on more than a one-time basis, at least in some regions and plans. Moreover, given the still-modest levels of HMO penetration, we can expect to see lower costs, and—relatively speaking at least—lower premiums as penetration levels increase in many communities.

But distinctions must still be made between lowering short-term prices and one-time costs, and lowering long-term system costs. The case that managed care can produce the former is rarely questioned today. The case that it can produce the latter is stronger than it was several years ago, but still open to question. The larger issues of ongoing technological advance and the nation's reluctance to address core ethical questions remain larger issues.

Managed Care: Quality and Consumer Satisfaction

When it comes to research on managed care quality and consumer satisfaction, much depends on the eye of the beholder. Survey findings appear to offer conflicting assessments; in many cases, the same data, depending upon interpretation, can reveal grave concerns regarding managed care or virtually no difference between managed care and indemnity plans.

Consumer Satisfaction

A review of studies on consumer satisfaction levels in managed care or fee-for-service suggests one overall finding: The great majority of insured individuals—in indemnity, PPO, or HMO plans—seem satisfied with their plan. One review concluded that fee-for-service plans scored slightly higher than HMOs on overall patient satisfaction surveys, but overall satisfaction scores generally range between 75 percent and 90 percent. On a survey taken by the Federal Employees Health Benefits Plan, for example, 86 percent of individuals in HMOs expressed satisfaction with their health plan overall (Group Health Association of America, 1995b).

On more specific measures, differences are more likely to emerge. HMOs generally will rate more highly on cost features, and sometimes on measures relating to preventive care; they will, not surprisingly, often score lower on measures relating to choice, access to specialists, or ease of getting an appointment.

Even in such subset areas, however, differences between managed care and fee-for-service plans are generally modest. On a particular index (for example, satisfaction with waiting times), managed care or fee-for-service may receive higher marks, and in some cases by as much as factors of three or four. But it is usually a case of 5 percent expressing dissatisfaction with one form, and 15 percent to 20 percent expressing dissatisfaction with another. In other words, at least 80 percent were satisfied in both types. For example, one recent study expressing concerns about managed care consumer satisfaction levels found that significantly greater numbers of managed care enrollees, (21 percent as opposed to 14 percent) rated their plan as poor or fair ("Warning Signs . . . ," 1995). The same study expressed concerns about the numbers of managed care enrollees rating their plans as poor or fair on a number of other specific indexes—but rarely did the dissatisfaction level (rating a plan poor or fair) rise above 25 percent.

Still another recent report, focusing only on nonelderly sick persons, also found that enrollees in managed care plans, while experiencing lower out-of-pocket costs, expressed higher levels of dissatisfaction on some measures. But here, too, the differences were fairly minimal, and the overall numbers hardly shocking. Fifteen percent of respondents in managed care plans, for example, reported that the time a physician spent with them was inadequate, as compared to 6 percent in fee-for-service plans. And 12 percent of enrollees in managed care plans (as opposed to 6 percent in fee-for-service plans) reported that their general physician failed to explain what he or she was doing ("Sick People . . . ," 1995). Again, while such numbers may reveal room for improvement, they hardly constitute cause for alarm.

Such a conclusion, however, requires one major modification. While high percentages of those in all types of plans tend to express general satisfaction, it must be recalled that, in any given year, most enrollees rarely have need to use their plan. When they have such need, it most commonly takes the form of a visit to a primary care physician they have chosen through some mechanism.

It is difficult to imagine how individuals seeking no or little care might be dissatisfied with service or care in their plans. In most consumer-satisfaction surveys, then, there may be a substantial bias toward reported satisfaction. There may be good reason, therefore, to weight such surveys toward those who have sought and received care.

Quality and Managed Care

The literature on the quality of care in managed care plans, and especially HMOs, is voluminous, and defies simple summation. But the weight of the evidence suggests—and virtually all systematic studies of quality in HMOs, especially in group and staff model HMOs—concludes that, as one reviewer put it, "Quality of care in HMOs is equivalent and sometimes better than under fee-for-service arrangements" (Shortell and Hull, 1994). "From over two decades of research studies," concluded another review, "there is convincing and consistent evidence that PGP (prepaid group) and staff-model HMOs reduce hospital use and overall cost relative to indemnity plans, while maintaining a level of service quality similar to that found in the FFS system" (Miller and Luft, 1993).

Newspapers, of course, are filled with anecdotes of care denied, and incentives imposed on physicians to withhold care. But studies, including the twelve-year RAND Corporation experiment, reveal that the reductions in utilization associated with managed care have not negatively affected the overall health status of managed care enrollees. Many have concluded, in fact, that much of the lower utilization reflects a reduction in unnecessary or inappropriate procedures. And multiple studies have revealed that enrollees in HMOs are more likely to be covered for a wide range of preventive services, including prenatal care, PAP smears, mammograms, clinical breast exams, and prostate examinations.

Consumer Satisfaction, Quality, and Managed Care

Overall, then, it appears that on the criteria of quality of care and consumer satisfaction, HMOs are performing at least as well as traditional fee-for-service plans.

Still, a number of striking caveats to such a conclusion stand out. Above all, the great majority of data, especially on measures of quality, comes from staff and group model HMOs. There is much less information on PPOs, IPAs, or POS plans, the managed care forms experiencing the greatest expansion in recent years. The absence of data on IPAs is particularly significant, because it is here (as we shall see in Chapter Two) that direct capitation of physicians may be most aggressive, and where physicians may be most at risk for higher utilization and costs. There is certainly some logic that if one were to seek out higher levels of consumer dissatisfaction or quality concerns, the aggressively capitated IPA plan might be the place to start.

Moreover, data on managed care consumer satisfaction and quality levels in the Medicaid and Medicare programs is spottier, both in terms of quantity of studies and consistency of findings. While a 1994 study by the American Hospital Association, for example, found beneficiaries in HMOs and in traditional Medicare to be equally satisfied with their quality of care (Group Health Association of America, 1995b), a Department of Health and Human Services Inspector General's survey detected significant levels of dissatisfaction on some measures among Medicare HMO enrollees ("Bad News About Medicare HMOs . . . ," 1995). Among other things, the report found that 43 percent of Medicare HMO enrollees surveyed had been asked (illegally) about their health status before enrolling. And while one comprehensive review concluded that quality in the Medicare and Medicaid HMOs was on a par with that in traditional forms, it also reported that the quality of care delivered in the Medicaid program overall was below that of private plans (Shortell and Hull, 1994).

There are also considerable concerns—based in part on logic, in part on anecdote, and in part on research—about the quality of HMOs in treating the chronically ill, especially the mentally ill. Managed care advocates can certainly outline why systems that are more integrated and have greater incentives to engage in prevention and to avoid high-cost episodes of care are particularly well-suited to managing and treating these higher-cost cases. But equally compelling logic can assert that capitated primary care physicians may be reluctant to approve adequate levels of specialty care, or that individuals with serious disabilities, especially mental disabilities, may be less able to aggressively assert their rights and opportunities in managed care settings. Not surprisingly, perhaps, the treatment of mental illness was the most documented exception to the overall finding that HMOs perform as well on quality as traditional insurance plans (Shortell and Hull, 1994).

Finally, a review of studies in consumer satisfaction and quality reveal significant concerns regarding continuity of care. One recent report, for example, found that nearly half the respondents in a nationwide survey had changed health care plans in the last three years, and that three-quarters of those did so involuntarily, mostly because their employers ceased offering coverage or they changed jobs ("Warning Signs . . . ," 1995). Such problems may be particularly acute in Medicaid managed care settings, where many recipients move in and out of health plans as they move in and out of welfare. As a result, it has been suggested, Medicaid managed care plans have generally failed to achieve preventive care objectives (Rosenbaum, 1995).

Such findings raise at least two related questions: First, to what extent do high plan turnover rates reduce incentives for delivering preventive care services? Second, do such high turnover rates and continuity concerns suggest a problem with a system in which employers, rather than individuals, choose insurance plans?

In commenting on these realities, one manager at the Intermountain HealthCare System, a Utah-based integrated system, noted that his system treats individuals as if they are enrolled for life (Brent James, interview, 1995). Certainly, such a view represents a healthy, public-spirited approach. It may even represent an accurate assessment of reality—in Utah. But in regions of the country where populations are more mobile, where job changes are more common, and where competing plans are more numerous (thereby increasing the probability that changing jobs means changing plans and physicians) treating someone for two to three years may be the more realistic expectation.

Overall, this is a scenario that has fostered some, most notably in Minnesota, to think more about individual rather than employer choice of plan, and more about that choice focusing not on an MCO or insurer, but on the specific delivery system from which an individual would receive care. Under such a system, changing jobs might have no impact on continuity of care.

Public Policy and Managed Care in the 1990s

The rise of managed care, and of the organizations delivering it, raises a number of public policy issues. The most controversial of these center on managed care's incentives to reduce utilization, and most particularly on means by which providers are paid. To many consumers, of course, such incentives remain synonymous with the means by which care may be denied. The result has been a series of consumer-protection proposals—some appropriate, some not—aimed at protecting consumers against some of the dangers inherent in the managed care construct.

Some of these proposals accept the values of managed care, and thus focus only on its potential excesses. Others—most notably any-willing-provider laws—go further, achieving what can be labeled *anti-managed-care* status. Proposals of both types will be reviewed in Chapters Eight and Nine. Physician payment strategies, and in particular the rise of capitation, will be discussed in Chapter Two, with policy issues relating to provider risk sharing discussed in Chapters Eight and Nine.

The anticipated extension of managed care to the Medicaid and Medicare programs has also raised a host of issues, most notably the potential of managed care to reduce government expenditures in these programs. The anticipation of a dramatic increase in enrollments of public beneficiaries in private managed care plans, however, may also have profound implications for the nation's safety net, which has survived intact largely due to the flow of funds from those programs. (These issues will be discussed in Chapter Ten.) Other significant public program issues include the capacity of states to monitor care in Medicaid managed care programs (Chapter Nine) and strategies for purchasing Medicare managed care products (Chapter Eight).

In a broader sense, the rise of managed care has set the stage for the restructuring—into larger, more organized units—of the nation's health care delivery system. As such, the rise of managed care is intricately related to the many policy issues flowing from that reorganization. Among other things, these include concerns about the maintenance of a competitive marketplace (Chapter Seven), the rise of for-profit provider and insurance organizations (Chapters Four and Ten), and the capacity of purchasers and consumers to compare price and quality in managed care plans (Chapter Eight).

Chapter Two

Sharing the Risk
Capitation and Other Strategies

Conventional wisdom reports that capitation is sweeping the nation. That wisdom is both right and wrong. If defined as the public would generally tend to define it—that is, the prepayment of a fixed amount of money to an HMO for delivery of a package of benefits— then the use of capitation is clearly expanding, and dramatically.

But as health care professionals are prone to define capitation, the nature of its national sweep is less apparent. Inside the health care beltway, capitation generally refers to a means by which health care providers, as groups or individuals, get paid. This can include, as in the public's definition of capitation, direct payments by an employer to an HMO. But it also includes payments from the HMO itself to a group or network of individual providers and to the payment by a group (for example, an IPA, a medical group, or a multispecialty clinic) receiving payments from an HMO to its individual providers.

If the subject is risk sharing, not just capitation, the complexity of payment definitions and mechanisms grows exponentially, for capitation is only one means of passing risk to providers. Today, payments to groups of providers or individual providers are increasingly likely to include some form of bonus, withhold, and/or risk pool. And not only are these more common but they are also appearing in greater variety and complexity. Indeed, some believe that the significance of capitation has been oversold, and that it is increasingly the case that—at the level of the individual provider especially—other forms of risk sharing are more significant and may be more likely to affect provider behavior and income.

Given these perspectives, the assumption that capitation, as a means of passing risk to providers, is sweeping the nation is part reality, part expectation, and part oversimplification. While direct capitation of groups and individual providers is clearly growing, and is generally expected to continue to grow, the trend—as well as the data to substantiate it—remains limited. Today it remains unclear what specific forms and directions capitation and other risk-sharing strategies may take.

But having attempted to put the trend or trends in place, it is also imperative to note at the outset that risk-sharing strategies may already have had an enormous impact on the organization of health care delivery. As we shall see, the concept of risk sharing by providers, its apparent ability to influence provider behavior, and the assumption that it will grow more common and prominent as a payment strategy, have combined to encourage the consolidation of providers into delivery systems that can seek and accept risk-sharing contracts. Such consolidation, aimed at producing greater coordination of care across a continuum of services, lower costs in care delivery (and thereby, presumably, great profit for capitated groups), and a capacity to assume responsibility for a larger share of the premium dollar, is a central component in the formation of new partnerships among insurers, hospitals, and physicians. For this reason, the concepts of capitation and risk sharing are absolutely central to the understanding of the ongoing reorganization of health care delivery today.

Capitation Today: An Overview

At present, the use of direct capitation of groups and individual providers remains a very small part of overall payments to health care providers. Surveys of providers, projecting that capitation revenues will constitute the vast majority of their business in 1996, may reflect rumor, even fear, more than reality. Providers, as a whole, still receive very little in capitated payments for treating Medicare and Medicaid recipients or from the uninsured. The great majority of PPOs (whether offered in insured or self-insured plans) pay providers on the basis of a discounted fee-for-service arrangement. So too, obviously, do those traditional indemnity insurance plans that still insure about one-third of those with employer-sponsored insurance.

Even within HMOs, as we shall see, payment of providers by capitation does not dominate over payment by salary or by discounted fee-for-service. Network and IPA HMOs may employ capitation (of groups and individual physicians) more than other means of paying primary care physicians. But most HMOs still pay specialists by discounted fee-for-service. Group and staff model HMOs are far more likely to pay salaries to all physicians (Gold and others, 1995). And hospitals are rarely paid via capitation, although they may be involved in other risk-sharing arrangements.

Thus, except in some (not all) very mature managed care markets, capitated payments comprise very small percentages of physician revenue. According to a late 1995 survey by *Medical Economics,* prepaid contracts represented just 15 percent of earnings of physicians who have such contracts (Walker, 1995). The modest level of revenues from capitated contracts is true even for medical groups—which are far more likely than independent physicians to be involved in capitated arrangements. Very few report high percentages of revenues in capitated payments. For example, in a study of capitation in multispecialty groups conducted by the Medical Group Management Association, only 36 percent of groups reported capitation revenues. And among these, such revenues represented just 20.5 percent of all revenues (David Gans, interview, 1995).

The most obvious exception to such a rule, of course, is California, where efforts to employ direct capitated arrangements have gone the furthest. According to one consultant, fifteen medical groups in California now report that 90 percent to 95 percent of their revenues come in capitated payments (P. Grant, quoted in Governance Committee, 1993).

Even in the far West, according to the Medical Economics survey, while 84 percent of physicians report PPO or HMO contracts, only 45 percent report having capitation income, amounting to just 23 percent of gross income (Walker, 1995).

Still, in the mid 1990s, it is clear that capitation payments to both primary care and specialty physicians are growing more commonplace. The trend clearly reflects a growing perception—to some a certainty—that placing groups and physicians at risk reduces utilization and lowers overall costs, thus enabling plans to lower premiums and reap greater profit.

There is also, according to many reports, a decline in the original and considerable reluctance of providers to accept the new payment mechanism. Once a cause of great financial uncertainty, increasing numbers of providers may be concluding that acceptance of capitation might be their most effective means of salvaging declining revenues and regaining control over larger amounts of the health care dollár, and reestablishing their control over the management of patient care.

There is no set scenario by which capitation strategies take hold in any given market. But the most likely pattern may be that direct capitation of individuals and groups begins to appear as markets reach about 20 percent HMO penetration, and as HMOs and other managed care plans begin to focus on competition with each other rather than with fee-for-service systems. (Direct capitation, reportedly, remains rare in markets with low managed care penetration.) At this point, perhaps, the perceived value of capitation as a tool in reducing utilization and costs, and thus premiums, takes on greater significance. Beginning with primary care physicians, the capitation strategy may spread to cover increasing numbers of specialists—and finally to all physician and hospital services.

Who's Being Capitated—and For What?

HMOs and the provider groups with which they contract employ a variety of capitation strategies, aimed at shifting different amounts of risk to different providers. However, research has produced only scanty data—mostly anecdotal—on the exact nature, extent, and impact of these strategies. Much of the problem stems from confusion over definitions and survey questions. Providers, for example, may say they are capitated, when in fact it is the medical group with which they are associated that is capitated, while they themselves are paid on a fee-for-service or salaried basis. HMOs may report they are capitating specialists because they have established a pool out of which specialists get reimbursed. But the pool of specialists, which controls the money, may be paying participants by discounted fee-for-service, with a withhold in case utilization and costs are higher than anticipated.

Researchers themselves sometimes add to the confusion. While focusing on capitation of individual physicians or small groups of physicians, they may emphasize the mechanism by which the individual provider is reimbursed. But when assessing the impact of capitation, defined more broadly, they may analyze integrated systems, such as a group model HMO or a multispecialty clinic, where the medical group is paid a fixed amount but where individual physicians mostly receive salaries. In a variety of circumstances then, whether or not individuals or groups of providers are capitated or not is largely a matter of definition, or degree, of perception. All of which makes it difficult to define capitated arrangements—and, as we shall see later, even harder to assess their impact.

Capitation for Primary Care Services Only

By all accounts, capitating the primary care physician or group for primary care only is still the most common capitation strategy. In perhaps the most comprehensive survey of capitation payments, conducted by Mathematica Policy Research, 57 percent of network/IPA models reported use of capitation as their primary means of paying individual primary care physicians (Gold and others, 1995). Table 2.1 shows some of the results of this survey. Group and staff models are more likely to pay by salary and are less likely to use capitation as their primary means of paying primary care physicians (Gold and others, 1995).

In its purest form, of course, capitating individual physicians or groups for primary care only may encourage primary care physicians to increase referrals to specialists, so as to reduce their risks and losses in higher-cost cases. For this reason, most plans invoking this capitation strategy will almost certainly add incentives—aimed at the group or the individual physician—in the form of withholds or bonuses structured to reduce referrals to specialists and admissions to hospitals. Thus, in this scenario, a primary care physician or group might receive a per-member-per-month payment equal to about 15 percent of the total premium, with a bonus or withhold arrangement (based in part on referrals to specialists) included that could raise or lower compensation.

Capitating for Full Professional Care

A more aggressive capitation strategy is to place primary care physicians at risk for both primary and specialty care services.

Table 2.1. Predominant Payment Method Used for Individual Primary Care Physicians, by Plan Type, 1994 (Percentage of Responding Plans).

Payment Method	All Plans (percent)	Group/ Staff (percent)	Network/ IPA (percent)	PPO (percent)
Fee For Service	43	3	37	93
With withholding or bonuses	12	0	24	3
With withholding or bonuses	31	3	12	90
Capitation	37	34	57	7
With withholding or bonuses	29	24	44	7
Without withholding or bonuses	8	10	12	0
Salary	19	62	6	0
With withholding or bonuses	11	34	4	0
Without withholding or bonuses	8	28	2	0
Number of plans	(107)	(29)	(49)	(29)

Source: Physician Payment Review Commission, 1995.

Under this scenario an individual or group of primary care physicians would receive a per-member-per-month (PMPM) payment amounting to about 40 percent of the premium dollar to cover all professional services. (Table 2.2 shows the allocation of the whole premium dollar in this sort of system.) The PMPM payment comes to perhaps $40 to $50 in California, and $45 to $55 in most other regions. Under such arrangements, obviously, primary care physicians may be at much greater risk depending in part on how much risk they, in turn, pass on to specialists, and how effective the primary care group is in monitoring and reducing specialty referrals and utilization. To reduce hospital costs,

Table 2.2. Division of the Premium Dollar (Percent).

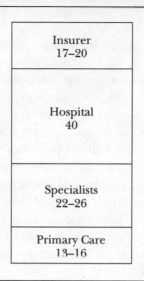

Insurer
17–20

Hospital
40

Specialists
22–26

Primary Care
13–16

generally paid by the HMO out of a different pool, the contracting HMO may build in incentives for the primary group to reduce hospital referrals and costs.

The increase of risk carried by primary care providers in such arrangements is, according to many, the reason such arrangements are particularly effective at lowering utilization of specialists and the procedures they order. The bearing of increased risk may also encourage primary care providers to improve practice efficiency via such means as implementing nurse triage arrangements, making more extensive use of alternative providers, and seeking assistance in practice management.

But placing primary care physicians at risk for more than their own services (some arrangements actually include a sizable element of risk-sharing for hospital services) may also be risky for the insurer and for the patient. Thus, the most potentially effective strategy (maximum risk) is also the most dangerous. The physician or group, especially when inexperienced in capitated arrangements, could easily underestimate, for example, the amount needed to pay specialists. Tracking mechanisms may not be adequate to report the amount owed to specialists, or the extent of what the insurance business calls *IBNR,* that is, incurred but not reported costs. The result can be serious financial shortages, leading either to inappropriate means of reducing costs (that is, undertreatment) or insolvency. The loser under these circumstances is likely to be the patient—or the insurer, who is still ultimately responsible. Not surprisingly, there have been multiple reports, especially from small medical groups in the Midwest, about physicians misjudging costs or accepting capitation rates that proved too low and suffering significant financial losses as a result (Terry, 1994b).

For these reasons, the full-professional-risk strategy is, according to most reports, now primarily invoked only with larger primary care groups, where risk can be more safely spread.

The full-professional-risk approach can also be undertaken by a multispecialty group. And since such groups have less need to contract for additional services outside the group, the multispecialty group may be better able to reduce financial risks, as well as spread them.

But whether invoked in a primary care or multispecialty group setting, capitation—especially when it involves larger numbers of services—encourages coordination and consolidation among providers. It may also highlight the need for (and enhanced value of) improving efficiency in practice management. In these ways, the expanded use of capitation, especially in the full-professional-risk form, drives increasing numbers of physicians toward larger and more complex organizational arrangements.

The Capitation of Specialists

For a variety of reasons, the age of specialty capitation has been slow in coming. For one thing, because capitation emphasizes incentives for reductions in referrals and procedures, it may be more threatening to specialists, who may remain resistant to a new paradigm in which raising income and profit is associated with doing less, and with raising the status and responsibilities of other—namely primary care—providers. For much the same reasons, when it comes to managing capitated contracts, primary care groups may prove superior to multispecialty groups, or at least those multispecialty groups organized and dominated by specialists. Such groups may be more reluctant to shift responsibility, status, and income to primary care physicians.

But in spite of the great emphasis on primary care physicians as the core element in the new ODS, the increasing use of specialty care risk-sharing strategies, even if slow in coming, is probably inevitable. It is specialists who direct most physician spending—perhaps twice that of primary care physicians. It is specialists who order the more expensive tests and procedures. It is specialists who direct most admissions to hospitals, where about 40 percent of health care dollars are spent. And, health services researchers have long argued, it is in reducing the overutilization of procedures, tests, and hospital admissions ordered and directed by specialists where the greatest potential savings are to be found.

As a result, if there is a growth industry in physician capitation, capitation of specialists may be it. While most specialty care, even in HMOs, is still paid for on a fee-for-service basis, the Mathematica survey found about 80 percent of HMOs reporting growing use of capitation for payment of specialists (Gold and others, 1995).

Not surprisingly, perhaps, the specialties most likely to be capitated are those entailing particularly high costs—cardiology and mental health. Indeed, psychiatrists rank right alongside pediatricians and family practitioners in terms of percentage of patient visits (23 percent) under capitation (Walker, 1995). As is the case with primary care physicians, specialty capitation may take a wide and increasing variety of forms. Specialists may be capitated directly by an HMO or by a primary care group with a full-professional-services contract. Capitation can be applied to the individual specialist, to all physicians in one specialty, or—as some report is more common today—to a network covering all specialty services. For example, CIGNA HealthCare in Florida reportedly capitates a network of specialists in part to enable broader geographic coverage, and in part because of the difficulty in managing and policing a large number of specialty capitation contracts (Terry, 1994a). Capitation of specialists as a network may also encourage coordination among them.

Alternatively, as is particularly prevalent in the coverage of mental health and substance abuse, HMOs or capitated groups may find it more efficient to contract or subcontract with carve-out firms that specialize in organizing and managing panels of specialty providers. The carve-out firm then assumes full-risk responsibility for providing services to plan enrollees in its specific area of service.

While data are scanty, these varieties of capitation strategies are reportedly producing considerable savings. CIGNA HealthCare in

Florida claims, for example, that capitating specialists has reduced outlays on spending for specialists by 30 percent. United Health-Care reports cost reductions of 15 percent to 40 percent when it shifts from fee-for-service to capitated payments ("Health Plans Force Changes . . . ," 1995), and *Medical Economics* reported that many HMOs are saving 10 percent to 20 percent by capitating specialists (Terry, 1994a). (Whether these savings are the result of lower payments to physicians, greater efficiencies in practice management and coordination, lower utilization by physicians, or some combination of the three is unclear.)

A Return of Fee-for-Service?

In keeping with industry standards, in which today's certain trend can be questioned tomorrow, some systems may be overturning the capitation tables, increasing their capitation of specialists while returning primary care physicians to fee-for-service arrangements.

This approach, which appears to look backward and forward at the same time, is reportedly being employed, for example, by United HealthCare in Minneapolis ("Health Plans Force Changes . . . ," 1995) and Pacific Physician Services of Redlands, California (Terry, 1995). Executives in these and other organizations find that paying primary care physicians by fee-for-service keeps primary physicians more contented, reduces incentives for referrals, is more satisfying to consumers, encourages more prevention, and doesn't penalize primary care physicians who may attract—by accident or otherwise—a higher-cost group of enrollees. Fee-for-service payments to primary care physicians may, Pacific Physician Services executives admit, increase payments for primary care and to primary care physicians. But the strategy may be cost effective in the long run, keeping patient enrollment up and primary care physicians committed to the system (Terry, 1995).

Moreover, applying the capitation strategy or salary to specialists focuses capitation on services where utilization and costs can be most dramatically reduced—that is, where the most money can be saved or lost. According to many reports, specialty capitation is likely to encourage specialists to assist primary care physicians in treating patients in lower-cost settings, and to inform primary care physicians when referrals that may once have seemed appropriate now seem unnecessary.

Whether or not such a strategy will spread remains unclear, as does the larger picture of specialty capitation. Theoretically, the excess of specialists may render them vulnerable to aggressive discounting strategies, reducing the need to invoke capitation. But cutting fees tends to induce higher rather than lower utilization. Just as important, it does little to encourage the long-term search for cost-effective medical practice, which is central to increasing profit in a capitated system.

Capitation of Hospitals

If the current logic of capitation suggests that it is a good idea to capitate specialists because that's where the savings are, that logic should hold true in spades for hospitals.

Yet while some consultants say hospital capitation is on the rise, it remains the exception rather than the rule—and the rare exception at that. In one 1994 study, only 25 percent of HMOs reported using capitation as a means of reimbursing any hospital services (Mitka, 1995). In another study, researchers found that just 7 percent of hospital revenues came in capitated payments (Fubini, 1996), with per diem payments being considerably more common. Even in Southern California, where capitated systems clearly dominate, only 40 percent of hospitals reported having any capitated contract (Kertesz, 1995).

Certainly, one reason behind the apparent reluctance of HMOs to capitate hospitals is that excess capacity weakens the hospital bargaining position, allowing HMOs—or medical groups with capitated contracts—to demand rock-bottom rates, sometimes well below those paid by Medicare. This leverage opportunity has been used with particular effect by California's fully capitated, large medical groups and IPAs. With many hospitals operating at less than 50 percent of bed capacity, few can reject contracts offered by groups controlling upwards of 200,000 lives, or even as few as 10,000.

The limited capitation of hospitals may also result from the limited control that hospitals have over admissions, and over the ordering of tests and procedures. These remain in the hands of physicians. Thus, physicians may remain the key focal point of capitation strategies. Indeed, as we have already seen, hospital utilization rates have already declined radically in competitive managed care markets, without hospitals themselves being directly capitated. From the MCO standpoint, then, capitating and otherwise providing incentives for physicians to reduce hospital utilization and costs may obviate the need to capitate the hospital itself.

Moreover, increasing numbers of HMOs and medical groups pay hospitals according to the diagnosis-related group system (or variations thereof) developed by Medicare. In this system, hospitals receive fixed payments based on the diagnosis of the case. Such a payment mechanism represents a form of capitation, giving hospitals incentives to limit costs in any particular case, although not necessarily in the aggregate. Hospitals may also participate in risk pool arrangements that create incentives to collaborate with physicians in controlling hospital utilization.

But in the case of hospital capitation, there may also be a larger strategic game at work. MCOs may be reluctant to capitate hospitals or the physician-hospital organizations (PHOs) they have formed because the insurers want to keep the savings from reductions of excess capacity and utilization for themselves. Capitating hospitals or PHOs might further reduce costs, but the savings would go to the hospitals and providers, not the MCO.[1]

An even more telling explanation for the limited capitation of hospitals may lie in the reluctance of MCOs to assist other organizations (such as large hospital-based systems) in the attempt to organize delivery systems capable of performing the full range of medical services and even insurance and utilization review functions. Such organizations would then be in a position to compete directly with the MCO, either by forming their own HMOs or by seeking direct contracts from employers. At minimum, such deliv-

---

[1]Such an analysis may run counter to economic theory, which would suggest that the minimum price that a hospital in a competitive marketplace will accept for a certain amount of service (providing it is risk neutral) should be the same, whether the hospital is paid by capitation or marginal cost of service. Capitation may lead to savings, but the savings could go either to the insurer or the hospital. (Savings would go primarily to the hospital, as insurers may fear, only if capitation rates were set too high.) The distribution of the savings, in any case, should be impervious to the form of payment.

ery systems might be able and willing to assume some of the functions (and the revenues that accompany their performance) now offered and controlled primarily by managed care companies. As one hospital authority noted, for example, MCOs made substantial investments in utilization review and management. Why, it may be asked, would they wish to turn that function over to a potential competitor? Utilization review, this analyst suggested, could soon become the MCOs' own unique excess capacity problem.

In a still broader challenge, the emergence of the ODS—capable of delivering the full range of care and of managing that care—could raise questions about the value added by managed care companies, and about why 15 percent to 20 percent of the premium dollar need be retained by the MCO for providing that questionable added value.

Growing Complexity in Risk-Bearing Strategies

Direct capitation is not the only form by which risk is transferred to providers. Today there is also a boom in incentives aimed at encouraging or discouraging various physician behaviors. In the Mathematica survey, for example, over 40 percent of HMOs reported making increased use of such incentives in paying both primary care and specialty physicians over the last three years (Gold and others, 1995).

Today, HMOs of all types are increasingly likely to alter physician payment amounts based on such criteria as patient satisfaction and outcomes, enrollee turnover rates, and quality measures, as well as the more traditional incentive measures of referral practices and utilization. According to the Mathematica survey, while utilization and cost measures are invoked most frequently, significant percentages of managed care plans (especially HMOs) are employing measures of quality (46 percent), patient complaints and grievances (49 percent), and consumer surveys (36 percent), as well as a variety of other measures (Gold and others, 1995). Table 2.3 sets out the range of utilization and cost measures in more detail.

Thus, for example, HealthPlus (an IPA model HMO in Maryland) includes immunization and mammogram rates as one of three elements in an incentive program that could boost a participating physician's income by as much as 15 percent ("Plans

**Table 2.3. Use of Selected Measures to Modify Primary Care
Physicians' Compensation, by Plan Type, 1994
(Percentage of Responding Plans).**

Measure to Modify Compensation	All Plans	Group/ Staff HMOs	Network/ IPA HMOs	PPOs
Consumer surveys	36	37	55	3
Quality measures	46	54	64	7
Patient complaints and grievances	49	57	61	21
Enrollee turnover rates	21	11	36	3
Provider productivity	24	43	26	3
Utilization or cost measures	57	50	74	34
Plans responding (number)	107	28	50	29

Note: As many as two plans did not respond to certain items. The sum of the percentages may be greater than 100 percent, because plans may use multiple measures.

Source: Physician Payment Review Commission, 1995.

Pay Doctors . . . ," 1995). And Kaiser Permanente in Southern California has considered a program in which physicians, based on group performance, may make up to $3,500 per year in bonuses related to hospital utilization, prescription of drugs, and patient satisfaction reports.

Not surprisingly, increased utilization of such incentives appears to be associated with higher levels of managed care penetration. This finding supports the contention outlined earlier that as managed care penetration increases, so, too, do physician risk sharing and the consolidation of provider groups designed to better spread risk and to improve access to the capitated dollar.

Given the nearly infinite number of potential risk-sharing arrangements (one consulting group mathematically calculated the figure to be somewhere over 421,000) (Governance Committee, 1994), it is virtually impossible to calculate the risk an individual physician or group may be bearing. The answer will depend on such factors as the proportion of overall business that is capitated, the amount and type of bonuses or withholds invoked, the services to which the capitation and risk-sharing arrangements apply, the amount of risk-sharing applied to the individual or to the group, and the use of contracts with other organizations to provide any of the services the group is contracted to provide.

It remains extremely difficult to reach beyond the aggregate numbers and anecdotes to see or measure the specific impacts of various forms of capitation. Thus, an analysis of a variety of studies and of an unlimited supply of anecdotal data may conclude that shifting risk to providers has an impact on provider behavior, and on utilization in particular. But in the end most research, and even most anecdotes, have not identified whether risk-sharing arrangements have an impact because employers are capitating HMOs, because HMOs are capitating groups or individuals, because groups are shifting risk to individual physicians, or most likely, because of some combination of all three.

The same type of problem emerges in trying to distinguish the impacts of the capitation from the perceptions of "being capitated." Overall, it may be fair to conclude that in terms of the capitation of individual physicians, rumor may be ahead of reality, and that perception of coming capitation is as much a market driver as the reality of capitation. But, in separating reality and perception, it is important to remember that physicians may not limit the concept of capitation to being personally at risk. They are very likely to associate being capitated not just with personal risk but also with their group being at risk, or with the HMOs with which they are contracting being at risk. When these associations are added into the capitation equation, the reality of rising capitation may begin to rival the perception.

Capitation and Quality

Just as unclear, and far more important ultimately, is the question of the impact of capitation and other forms of risk sharing on the quality of care delivered. The fast-disappearing world of fee-for-service may have put a value on overutilization, resulting in a price that increasing numbers of purchasers—employers and consumers— could no longer tolerate. Provider risk sharing, by contrast, raises the legitimate concern of underutilization or underservice, as physicians may face conflicts of interest between personal economic stakes and what may be best for the patient.

As discussed in Chapter One, there is not yet any systematically collected evidence suggesting that managed care and the risk-sharing strategies it employs do result in underservice or poorer quality of care overall. But such a conclusion hardly implies that the conflict doesn't exist or that significant instances of underutilization or service don't occur. Indeed, such instances may be most likely to occur where underservice would be most dangerous—among the highest-cost and often most vulnerable patients. (The greatest concerns about quality and managed care, it will be recalled, were expressed with regard to the mentally ill.)

It is also instructive to recall, as noted earlier, that the form of capitation viewed by many as most powerful in terms of lowering utilization is that of capitating an individual provider or small group of providers for a broad range of services. Yet such capitation is also likely to raise the greatest potential physician conflicts and pose the greatest risk to patients. It is certainly a positive sign, therefore, that anecdotal evidence indicates that the utilization of this capitation strategy remains limited and may be declining. These issues will be explored in greater detail in Chapter Eight.

The Logic of Full-Risk Capitation

For an increasing number of consultants, academics, and practitioners, the logical end game of capitation is the acceptance of full-risk capitation by an ODS. Indeed, today's efforts to organize such systems, whatever their form or leadership source, all have at their core the goal of efficiently coordinating care across a full spectrum of services and thereby increasing potential to compete for capitated contracts in which the ODS will be responsible for most or all of the services to be delivered.

The increasing acceptance of the ODS construct comes in part from clinical and organizational experience. As reviewed earlier, studies of staff and group model HMOs, which operate as integrated systems under such full-risk contracts, have demonstrated a capacity to reduce utilization of specialists and hospital services (Shortell and Hull, 1994; Miller and Luft, 1993).

Equally striking, if not even more so, has been the performance of California's large medical groups. These function very differently from traditional staff or group model HMOs. In contrast with those models, the California medical groups feature a nonexclusive relationship between HMOs and the groups with which they contract, more geographic dispersion of physician services, more direct risk sharing by physicians, and more reliance on flexible and contractual (as opposed to employment and ownership) relationships between the HMO and the medical group.

Today, presentations at conferences on changing health care markets are often dominated by data relating to the performance of these groups, much of it revealing overall cost declines of 25 percent or more, resulting in premiums that may be 20 percent to 30 percent lower than those in much of the rest of the country.

In spite of such evidence, the case for the inevitable joining of ODSs and full-risk capitation may remain more one of logic than of conclusive systematic analysis. But the logic is compelling, and the apparent economic imperative appears strong enough to be a major driver of current consolidation efforts. Capitation, the logic suggests, compels consolidation and organization of providers—to extend geographic coverage, to improve coordination of care, to reduce utilization, to improve efficiency, and to spread risk. It sharply elevates the value of lowering costs and thus the value both of improving efficiency and management of medical services and of instituting superior information systems that can transmit clinical and other data across a complex system. Finally, in its full-risk mode especially, capitation places a premium on coordination of medical services so as to yield lower costs overall, as opposed to lower costs for a given service (for example, primary care), which may result in higher costs for another service (for example, specialty services).

Each of these attributes, requirements, or challenges is a hallmark of the new ODS. Thus, the ascendancy of capitation—be it a fixed payment to a plan, a group, or a physician—is inextricably tied to, and is a major cause of, the emerging concept of the ODS.

POS Plans, Integration, and Capitation

All of which is not to conclude, however, that trends in risk sharing today will necessarily be the realities of risk sharing tomorrow. Indeed, it is possible to argue that a number of forces or aspects of ODSs could change the role of risk sharing in the new paradigm.

For one thing, it would appear that two of the strongest current marketplace trends—growth of POS plans, and capitation of individual physicians and groups—run counter to each other. The first offers the choice to go out of network; the second suggests that physicians or groups of physicians accept more direct responsibility for the costs of patient care.

But physicians cannot accept such responsibility without commensurate control over spending. Thus, if the POS option continues to gain public support and if consumers make substantial use of it, the option could pose an impediment to risk-sharing strategies. This would be particularly true if the individuals making the greatest use of the POS option prove to be those with high-cost conditions. Just when the capitated physician or group found themselves at greatest risk, they would have the least control.

Excluding out-of-network spending from the capitation payment does not, it should be emphasized, solve the problem. For one thing, such a strategy might encourage capitated providers to encourage high-cost cases to seek care elsewhere, a clearly unacceptable outcome. But even if the providers are both ethical and conscientious, the out-of-network option will leave them vulnerable. Imagine the scenario, for example, in which a patient with asthma seeks additional out-of-network care. But after treatment ordered by the out-of-network provider, the condition worsens, and the patient returns to the network. Hospitalization that the capitated physician thinks might have been avoided could be the first result.

To date, at least, anecdotal information suggests that such conflicts may remain more theoretical than actual, and most MCOs do not appear to be overly concerned about the potential conflict. To address such concerns, should they become significant, plan organizers might consider creation of a reinsurance mechanism to protect individual providers at risk, or establishment of a risk pool to cover all capitated providers for out-of-network services (Gold and others, 1995).

In addition to the POS issue, it is clear that some forms of organized systems may find capitation of individual physicians or small groups to be inappropriate or unnecessary. For example, if the system is highly integrated, including exclusive arrangements in which the provider works only for the system, capitation of the system as a whole may seem far more critical and relevant than capitation of the parts. This might be especially true if physicians held equity shares in the system. In such circumstances, all might be more focused on the productivity of the system as a whole. Capitation focused on the parts might be inappropriate, or more complicated than productive.

The same conclusion might result where a system deployed increasingly sophisticated information and data systems to select only those physicians who embraced conservative practice styles. Capitating such physicians would probably have, at best, a very modest impact. At worst, it would generate higher administrative costs and ill will, with no clear benefit.

In such circumstances, while risk sharing and capitation in particular may have been critical to the formation of organized systems, they may also prove less valuable once that system is operational. For these and other reasons, while direct capitation of providers may be a powerful driving force behind the ODS movement, its continuing growth once those systems are created and functioning is more problematic. There will then, after all, be a new system in place—and new strategies may seem more appropriate.

Risk Sharing and Public Policy

The increase in the utilization of risk-sharing strategies, like the rise of managed care in general, has raised a variety of public policy questions. These center on consumer protection in capitated systems, including grievance procedures in the face of denial of care and rights to know about financial relationships between HMOs, medical groups, and individual providers. These are discussed in Chapter Nine.

The rise of various risk-sharing strategies (and of the ODSs they have helped to spawn) has also led to increased interest in direct contracting (on a capitated basis) between employers and providers. Such contracting raises a complex web of quality, consumer protection, cost, and insurance regulation issues. These are discussed in Chapters Seven, Eight, and Nine.

Above all, perhaps, the rise of risk-sharing strategies has raised issues of the impact of those strategies on quality of care, and of means by which capitation may work to improve rather than threaten high quality in care delivery. These issues, too, are discussed in Chapter Eight.

Part Two

Uneasy Partnerships: Vulnerabilities and Opportunities in the New Marketplace

Chapter Three

Goals and Strategies in the Age of Managed Care

For health care professionals and MCOs the new competitive environment is marked by seemingly unprecedented levels of uncertainty and volatility. For many, especially some physicians and some hospitals, the primary result may be a growing sense of vulnerability. For some, especially larger MCOs and organizers of systems, the new environment may appear (however uncertain and precarious) laden with new opportunities. For still others, especially primary care physicians, vulnerability and opportunity may coexist.

A Fast-Changing Environment

For providers especially, the new marketplace realities (or at least the perception of fast-approaching new realities) often strike with considerable suddenness and force. Providers are either experiencing or expect to be experiencing a significant increase in the utilization of managed care strategies—including varieties of risk sharing. Where it has occurred, the replacement of cost-plus, fee-for-service medicine by a new paradigm featuring more price-sensitive purchasers choosing among larger and more organized prepaid health plans is placing an unprecedented squeeze on prices, costs, and profits. In growing numbers of markets, aggressive competition on price (at all levels of the delivery and insurance systems) is now an accepted fact. So, too, is the growing awareness of excess capacity, and of the increasing ability of health plan and system organizers to extract lower charges from providers willing to accept less revenue in order to attain more security.

Where new realities or paradigms have not yet set in, they are expected. Thus, whether driven by real or anticipated changes, MCOs, hospitals, and physicians are plotting new courses, which often means looking for new relationships and partners.

In the early stages of the current transformation, these and other realities of the changing health care marketplace are often met by rejection, resentment, or fear. Ultimately, however, a level of acceptance sets in, which can in turn generate new organizational efforts to at minimum maintain turf—and at maximum seize new opportunities for leadership and profit. Virtually all involved recognize threats to past position and future. But whether driven by fear or opportunity, the result has been a rush to restructure the health care delivery and insurance systems.

Consolidation, Profits, and New Partnerships

According to most analysts, the economic magnitude of the stakes is nothing less than massive. By some estimates, the numbers of individuals in HMOs could grow to over 110 million, including perhaps 25 million enrollees from the Medicare and Medicaid programs by very early in the twenty-first century. Given that Medicare premium growth may run three or four times that of commercial premiums, the premiums paid to HMOs could increase by over $150 billion between 1995 and 2000 (Hodapp and Samols, 1994).

Today it is widely assumed that such rapid growth (and the opportunities for profit for those properly positioned to take advantage of it) are leading what many have called our current cottage industry, consisting largely of independent providers, toward widespread consolidation of organizations, resulting in fewer, larger, more powerful, and (it is to be hoped) more efficient competitors. Predictions of a shrinkage in the numbers of HMOs from over 550 to somewhere between 200 and 300 are commonplace, and even if numbers are not reduced that dramatically, there is little doubt that trends toward larger market share for smaller numbers of HMOs will continue. On the hospital side as well, there are expectations of soaring numbers of hospital mergers and growing clout of larger and larger hospital systems. Thus, the emergence of a new marketplace in which larger, more integrated ODSs (defined, admittedly, in a multitude of ways) compete for managed care contracts and premiums is viewed as something close to inevitable.

Few expect the restructuring process (which in many markets is less extensive than insider journals proclaim) to be orderly. And while many express certainty as to the particular ability of one form or another of organization to survive, most such predictions are grossly premature.

Still, there has been and will continue to be a dramatic increase in the formation of partnerships (including mergers and acquisitions), often featuring new relationships or changes in long-established relationships. Physicians are forming MCOs, MCOS and hospitals are purchasing physician practices, and MCOs are consolidating at a rapid pace. Hospitals are merging and forming strategic alliances with former competitors. Physicians and hospitals are attempting to bridge decades of distrust and form PHOs; new entities are emerging to manage physician practices or relationships between physicians, hospitals, and MCOs; and even the most venerable of institutions—Kaiser Permanente, the Mayo Clinic, and many of the nation's most prestigious academic medical centers are finding that they must adjust or suffer serious consequences.

Studying Market Change: A Challenge All Its Own

The study of these changes has been anything but easy. For one thing, the new relationships vary across a wide range of criteria—by who's leading, by types of markets, by levels of consolidation or integration sought. Analysis is further complicated by the reality, as noted earlier, that rumor and anecdote are far more plentiful than systematic analysis, or even solid case studies. In such circumstances, a handful of successful experiments can become an inexorable trend, at least in the eyes of those potentially affected.

In fact, much less may be going on than meets the eye. For example, fee-for-service payment to individual physicians still lingers, and may continue to thrive in many circumstances. But, from the perspective of physicians, hospitals, MCOs, and other actors, waiting to find out what's working and what isn't or what is actually happening and what is not may involve waiting too long.

Research is further complicated by limitations in terminology and in distinctions between types of organizations. As organizational forms adjust, long-standing distinctions—as between IPA, network, and group model HMOs—break down. Consider, for example, the case of a large medical group, dispersed over a number of sites, using a combination of member physicians and independent physicians with whom it has contracts to service a full-risk managed care contract. Is it a medical group? an IPA? And what type of HMO do we call the organization that may be contracting with it and other similar groups to provide care?

Lastly, there may be confusion over concepts of consolidation and integration. Some analysts seem to refer to virtually all efforts to bring organizations together as integration. Others seem more prone to restrict the term to mean increasing coordination within a system, making parts of the whole work better. (Webster's, interestingly, doesn't help, defining both integration and consolidation as "joining together into one whole.") Webster's notwithstanding, however, the distinction is probably an important one. On the whole, consolidation in health care systems has come more easily than integration, and some forms of integration (clinical especially) have been harder to achieve than others.

In this and the following chapters we shall explore how MCOs, hospitals, and physicians are adjusting organizationally to a changed and changing environment: the goals they may seek and the strategies they must pursue; their assets and liabilities in that pursuit; the new organizational relationships that are emerging from those pursuits; and how all these efforts fit into their image of a role in the organized delivery system of the future.

Two Overarching Goals

Obviously, in a volatile marketplace, hospitals, MCOs, and physicians will have needs and goals that vary with a multitude of factors, including the extent of managed care penetration in a marketplace, the numbers of hospital systems that may be present in a market, and the presence or lack thereof of organized medical groups.

Still, it may be possible to identify broad goals upon which nearly all must focus—and to an increasing extent do appear to be focusing. These we define as pursuit of access to and control over the premium dollar, especially the capitated premium dollar, and pursuit of proper positioning to lead, be essential to, or function productively in the emerging breed of ODSs.

Focusing on the Premium Dollar

Central to marketplace restructuring are the efforts of individuals, groups, and organizations to guarantee themselves or their organizations access to or more control over revenues associated with managed care contracts.

The logic of this emphasis flows, in large part, from the "that's where the money is" principle—or in this case, where the money is expected to be. Increasingly today, unlike the not-too-distant past, guarantees of revenue (and patients) require affiliation with an MCO. Solo physicians find that their ex-patients are now *covered lives* in an MCO—and thus out of reach. Specialists and hospitals find that referrals come increasingly through networks and panels, and not necessarily from reputation or decades-long associations with other physicians.

Closely related to the "that's where the money is" principle is what might be called the Wall Street principle—the perception and reality of where profit lies. In a health care system laden with excess capacity and perceived inefficiency and in an environment where many believe that capitation and other managed care strategies can significantly lower costs, the ability to make a profit is often linked to the ability to control more of the premium dollar. The general contractor—the one who controls the inevitable restructuring, reorganizing, and right-sizing—will have the best opportunity to profit. And, generally speaking, the more control exerted over more parts of the system—physicians, hospitals, other professional services, and insurance functions—the greater that opportunity.

A focus on the premium dollar entails, in large part, a focus on the traditional goals of market share and power. But it also provides an instructive and relevant emphasis on the meaning of market share in the managed care context. In that context, market share is not determined simply by percentages of covered lives an organization may control: it is also a matter of how much of the covered life—primary care, specialty care, hospital care, even insurance functions—an organization controls.

Focusing on the ODS

One might argue that repositioning an organization to assume a more prominent role in the ODS is but a part of the larger goal of securing access to and control over the premium dollar. But the two goals entail different emphases. Almost by definition, the ODS concept places particular focus on organizational efforts that are particularly relevant to the delivery of care. Thus the literature on the ODS emphasizes integration of clinical services and of physicians in the larger system. It stresses the efficient coordination of care over a broad continuum of medical services, and a capacity to improve and demonstrate high quality. And (at least according to most definitions) it draws attention to health status of a defined population, prevention strategies to improve that status, and means of measuring and competing on it.

As will be noted later, the great majority of organized systems— even those capable of accepting full capitation—are probably far from achieving the goals (especially the quality and clinical goals) established by themselves or others. To date, most are likely to be more focused on bringing the pieces of an organization together than on making them work more productively. Still, the ODS construct is a critical one in today's marketplace. Even if hopes for the elevation of clinical and quality considerations fall short of targets, the construct is expected to remain central to marketplace reconstruction.

Strategies to Achieve the Goals

Given these overriding goals, and recognizing that strategies to achieve them will vary by market, size of organization, and a multitude of other factors, what are the major strategies that MCOs, hospitals, and physicians must consider in pursuit of these goals?

Although few lists can be either exclusive or exhaustive, it may be valuable to outline the strategies for controlling premium dollars and positioning actors for a role in the ODS that seem most prominent in today's marketplace. Such an effort should help put the organizational and other efforts of MCOs, hospitals, and physicians in context.

- *Increase market power by making an organization and its affiliates more indispensable and influential.* Achievement of this objective will, in general terms, enable a group to purchase for less and sell for more. At minimum, this may mean increasing the size or market share of an organization and thus its capacity to compel others to include it in networks or service contracts. Thus MCOs may merge, in part to increase their numbers of covered lives—and consequently their leverage in extracting lower prices from providers. Hospital systems may expand to render their inclusion mandatory in an MCO network or system. Hospitals may form PHOs in an attempt to bind physicians to them—thus, among other things, increasing their ability to force MCOs seeking contracts with those physicians to contract with the hospital as well.

- *Expand the capacity of the organization to enable it to do what it couldn't do before, including expansions of products offered and services covered.* At minimum, this may entail achieving enough geographic reach to accept capitated contracts in a region. Medical groups or clinics may, therefore, merge with others or expand geographically, and also cover more services. In a more aggressive vein, expansion may entail the development of new capacities to perform functions generally performed by others. Physicians might either form an HMO, enabling them to secure managed care contracts directly, or purchase outpatient facilities to control services once offered and controlled by hospitals. Large health systems might merge or expand geographically so as to seek contracts directly from self-insured employers, bypassing insurers.

Additionally, new and expanded positioning might include increasing the numbers of health care or other products offered. Among other things, such a strategy will enable an MCO to offer one-step shopping to large employers, whereby an employer could offer several products to employees while contracting with only one insurer. Thus, a staff or group model HMO might offer a new PPO product, either marketing it directly, or renting it out to other insurers or to self-insured employers. An MCO might offer a new workers' compensation product or a women's services product, or it might expand its offerings in specialty carve-outs. A health plan or hospital might develop and market a physician management organization or an information system. Such product expansions can take advantage of economies of scale, generate greater revenues, and offer one-stop shopping to purchasers.

• *Increase capacity to accept capitated contracts.* In addition to requiring comprehensive efforts to reduce costs, achievement of this objective may necessitate, among other things, a focus on securing services of primary care physicians, on broadening a network to offer enough choice of physicians to potential enrollees, on enhancing capacities to spread and manage risk, and on improving physician management systems. Thus medical groups may merge to safely spread risk or accept more capitated contracts. Hospitals or MCOs may purchase or secure long-term relationships with primary care physicians. Medical groups may seek management or capital assistance from a physician management organization.

• *Improve administrative performance, increase efficiency, generate economies of scale, and reduce duplicative costs.* Almost any organization will seek these objectives, but they require special focus in an industry presumed to be highly inefficient, and where organizations are expanding rapidly in size, scope, and diversity of products offered. Hospitals may undertake joint ventures, partnerships, or full mergers. Physicians may seek to reduce administrative costs by forming larger groups or participating in management services organizations. MCOs may merge to spread costs of information and administrative services over a larger enrollee base.

• *Improve information systems necessary to coordinate and integrate new, larger, and more complex systems and to assist in integration.* Improved efficiency in both administrative and clinical functions will require improved information technology and services. Such services will be required to track patients over the continuum of care, assist in selecting physicians and monitoring physician output, and improve efficiency of clinics and physician practices.

• *Secure access to capital.* Technically, securing access to capital may be more a tactic than a strategy, in that it is clearly a means more than an end. But it is absolutely central to most partnering strategies, especially when expansion or consolidation appears to be an imperative. In the changing marketplace, almost all provider organizations are assuming they must grow, merge, or sell. (Even those who may wish to downsize—by closing a hospital or by selling a physician group to focus on insurance services—will want to grow in their chosen area of focus.) Almost all such growth will require capital, often in large amounts; so, too, will new information and management systems. Physician groups may seek capital to start their own HMOs or expand information services; hospitals or MCOs may require capital to purchase physician practices; MCOs will need capital to expand to new markets—either by organizing new networks there or by acquiring existing ones.

- *Improve clinical performance and ability to compete on quality of care.* Higher quality, it is hoped, will increase market power, making delivery systems more attractive to MCOs, and all organizations more attractive to purchasers. Thus, HMOs and other ODSs may invest in clinical information systems, develop and implement protocols and clinical guidelines, or study variations in physician practice and outcomes. An MCO or hospital chain may contract or otherwise ally with a prestigious hospital or clinic.

Many of these strategies are compatible, even overlapping. But conflicts can exist. The rush to expand can clash with the need to integrate or improve efficiency. Limitations on available capital may force choices between, for example, investments in physician practices and in new information systems. Efforts to improve long-term positioning on quality may not draw adequate attention from top executives focused on more immediate crises relating to mergers, acquisitions, or other short-term market power and market share concerns.

Even more obvious is the reality that any given organization may need to emphasize some strategies over others, and invoke different strategies in different markets. Nevertheless, the list may help serve as a guidepost in the exploration of the needs and partnering activities of the various major players.

Two Final Questions

As noted earlier, the concept of the ODS encompasses a variety of definitions and forms. But two elements of its original formulation may be particularly worthy of note, one because it is the focal point of much strategic planning today, the other because it may have critical implications for the pursuit of quality.

Ownership or Contractual Relationships: How Much Integration?

At any "Changing Health Care Markets" conference in 1992 or 1993, it was almost inevitable that some presenter would offer a slide or overhead chart depicting a matrix of emerging health care systems. Vertical and horizontal axes in the matrix might represent different variables on different presenters' slides, but in the top right-hand corner would be something labeled the "fully integrated health care system," or the "organized" or "integrated health care system." The outcome of the churning marketplace, of the rise of managed care, and of the kinds of strategic efforts outlined earlier in this chapter, it would be argued, lead ultimately to higher levels of integration—horizontal and especially vertical—in health care systems.

The more integrated system, in which major delivery system components were both consolidated and integrated into one organized system, usually including the insurance component, was widely presumed to be capable of producing the greatest value, and to be best adapted to accepting managed care contracts and responsibility for providing the full continuum of care for defined populations. Such systems could come in a number of forms: staff and group model HMOs; health care systems that included several hospitals and clinics and offered varieties of managed care products; even large multispecialty groups with strong management styles, high levels of physician commitment, and long-term relationships with hospitals.

But whatever the particular style or structure of the system, it seemed to be widely presumed that when it came to integration, more was generally better. Additionally, ownership generally seemed to be preferable to contractual relationships—which, almost by definition, could not achieve some key goals of integration.

Today, as organizations adopt various market strategies and pursue various levels of integration, there may still be considerable consensus on what constitutes integration in delivery systems. There may even be considerable consensus on the logic of integration—that more integration is more likely to achieve some of the goals postulated.

But there is much more doubt regarding the value of those goals, and on whether or not some of them might be achievable via less integrated forms, especially forms that may seek less vertical integration. Most specifically, many now argue that contractual relationships between MCOs, hospitals, and physicians (even between separate groups of primary care and specialty physicians), properly structured, can achieve many of the advantages of employment or single-ownership systems without taking on the disadvantages—including reduced flexibility and heavy commitments of capital to facilities and staff—that generally mark those systems.

Thus the growing popularity of so-called virtual integration constructs.

We shall return to this division—which should not be exaggerated, as almost all now recognize middle ground—in Chapter Six.

The Issue of Quality

Early discussions of integrated systems also featured—as most discussions still do today—an emphasis on clinical integration, on improving coordination of care over a full continuum of services. The capacity to improve the quality of care delivered—defined as much more than a reduction in utilization and cost—was viewed as a hallmark, perhaps even the raison d'etre of the integrated system.

Consequently, those promoting and even just anticipating the arrival of the integrated system highlighted such features as taking responsibility for a defined population; focusing on health status and prevention; and improving physician integration, that is, the commitment of the physician to the larger organization; and aligning incentives within the delivery system. All of which appeared to be patient centered, and quality centered, including the underlying, implicit assumption that more integrated systems would produce higher quality at a lower price, and thereby higher value.

Such a focus was, perhaps, not surprising. To academics and policy-oriented thinkers, clinical progress and higher quality were natural points of emphasis. For employers, especially the large businesses that often promoted the ODS concept, the assumption that higher quality (as opposed to lower price) would be the driving force and goal in the new marketplace was also a comfortable one.

But the rapidly evolving health care marketplace is directing the attention of ever-larger business entities to huge amounts of revenue and potential profit. Today, those entities are primarily focused on right-sizing, new partnering relationships, economies of scale, market leverage and selection, securing access to managed care revenue flows, and marketing more products.

Just where quality fits in is less clear. Admittedly, purchasers may be more demanding, especially in demanding value, generally defined as quality divided by price. But price is a tangible factor, and in today's market, very susceptible to downward pressure. Quality, by contrast, is harder to define, and perhaps more difficult to improve and demonstrate (especially if price must be reduced). Thus, it may be easier today to raise value by lowering price rather than by raising quality. It may, then, be reasonable to question how the goal of improving quality will fare in a marketplace so sensitive to price and profit. The movement toward clinically integrated delivery systems featuring competition on quality as well as price may have a logical ring. But its inevitability, at least in the short run, is unproven. This subject, too, shall be revisited.

In the following three chapters we review the nature of the new partnerships between MCOs, hospitals, and physicians. Chapter Four looks at the nature and extent of consolidation efforts within each sector—generally referred to as *horizontal* integration. Chapter Five reviews efforts to create new relationships between the three actors—especially those efforts geared to securing relationships with primary care providers—generally referred to as *vertical* integration. Chapter Six reviews the construct of the ODS, the issues that construct is raising, and the position of each set of actors to lead in the formation and direction of those systems.

Chapter Four

First Steps
The Strategy of Consolidation

Inherent in key strategic objectives of all major actors is the assumption that growth, even survival, in the new marketplace means forming new partnerships, expanding them, and improving their performance. Such partnerships, as we have noted, can entail both horizontal integration (consolidation within each sector—physicians, hospitals, and MCOs) and vertical integration, featuring relationships across sectors.[1]

Generally speaking, horizontal consolidation has proven easier to achieve, and has been more dramatic in scope and impact. It is also true that, with the possible exception of the needs of MCOs and hospitals to secure ties to primary care physicians, horizontal partnerships have been a higher priority for most actors. This may suggest that the goals of market share and power, more closely associated with horizontal consolidation, may be the strongest market drivers. It is for this reason that these relationships have drawn the most scrutiny from antitrust enforcement agencies.

Generally speaking also, vertical integration—especially at the clinical level—has proved more difficult to achieve. Moreover, as discussed in Chapter Three, the nature of the vertical relationships required has undergone more serious questioning, with many

---

[1]Analysts employ different definitions for horizontal and vertical integration. Since we are focused on physicians, hospitals, and MCOs, our definition defines relationships within each of these sectors as horizontal. Other analysts might disagree, considering, for example, integration between primary care physicians and specialists as vertical integration.

organizations focusing more on contractual relationships (which may still achieve virtual integration or something close to it) rather than more formal ownership relationships. Here again, however, a key exception may lie in the need of MCOs and hospitals to cement ties with physician groups, especially primary care groups.

Consolidation in Managed Care: The Big Get Bigger

Consolidation among MCOs, especially in more mature markets, has been nothing less than dramatic. Continuation of this trend, including its extension to less mature markets, is viewed as nearly inevitable. Mergers or acquisitions of organizations are perceived as fueling mergers and acquisitions of competing organizations. All of which may involve new waves of such activity, undertaken by organizations that are themselves the results of earlier consolidations.

Examples are numerous:

- Aetna is acquiring U.S. Healthcare for about $9 billion, creating the nation's fourth largest HMO and the single largest medical benefits company, which will cover twenty-three million Americans.
- Minnesota-based United HealthCare (UHC) recently acquired MetraHealth (a company resulting from a merger of the health care organizations of Travelers Insurance and Metropolitan Life). UHC provides full medical coverage for four million individuals and specialty coverage for millions more. MetraHealth has just over ten million members ("Sick People in Managed Care . . . ," 1995).
- Humana has acquired Empheses Financial Group. With the acquisition, Humana will have premium revenues of about $5.5 billion. Empheses was the tenth largest commercial group health insurer ("Medpartners & Mullikin to Merge," 1995).
- Harvard Community Health Plan and Pilgrim Health Care have merged, demonstrating that nonprofits have been active on the consolidation front as well. The two have arranged to acquire a third HMO, based in New Hampshire.

Such activity is not—at least not yet—producing a significant reduction in the number of managed care firms. Overall, the number of HMOs alone (excluding other forms of managed care plans) has declined modestly, to just under 600, after peaking at about 650 in 1987 (Group Health Association of America, 1995a). But the big are getting bigger, with increasing numbers of enrollees and revenues moving into a shrinking number of dominant organizations.

Thus, the market share of the larger MCOs is rising. In 1991, the largest twenty HMOs had 33 percent of total enrollees—12.9 million individuals (Group Health Association of America, 1992). Just three years later, that percentage had soared to 57 percent—29 million individuals—and that was prior to a number of 1995 mergers and Aetna's 1996 aquisition of U.S. Healthcare (Group Health Association of America, 1995a).

Many anticipate that the number of MCOs may continue to decline to somewhere between two and three hundred, primarily as weaker organizations with less than 100,000 enrollment are acquired by larger ones who see acquisition as an easier vehicle for expansion into new markets than seeking to build networks from the ground up. Given some projections of managed care growth, the average-size MCOs might then soar in the next five years from 150,000 members and average revenues of $300 million to 1.5 million members with average revenues of $3.5 billion (Hodapp and Samols, 1994).

Many also anticipate that consolidation will not only reduce the overall number of HMOs, but—perhaps far more important from a marketplace competition point of view—the numbers competing in each market as well. Without question, any review of maturing managed care markets—most notably Minneapolis and Southern California—suggests such a probability.

Even this trend, however, may have some limits, especially in the short run. Most notably, the rise of Medicaid and Medicare managed care and the resultant opening of major new managed care markets may keep interest in market entry high, at least in those markets where enrollment of public program recipients is expected to be particularly large.

Additionally, it must be noted that consolidation of MCOs does not always come easily. Indeed, the most heralded consolidation of 1995 proved to be no consolidation at all. The announced merger of the California Blue Cross affiliate, Wellpoint Health Networks, and Health Systems International (a result of a previous merger between Qualmed and Health Net) would have created a company with over $6 billion in revenues, over 4 million members in HMOs and PPOs, and over 8 million in specialty product plans such as pharmacy, and dental ("The Race to Consolidate," 1995). By the end of the year, however, the merger effort had disintegrated.

Who's Getting Bigger

In viewing such rapid consolidation, it is impossible to ignore the reality of who is getting bigger. They are, on the whole, national versus locally based and independent plans; commercial insurers; and, most striking of all, for-profit versus nonprofit insurers.

While these trends are distinguishable, they are also related and in some ways additive. Taken together, they pose the prospect of an industry increasingly dominated by large, for-profit national enterprises, alarming some who fear not just a loss of competition but a loss of community control and charitable ethic as well.

The Rise of For-Profit Health Plans

The greatest growth in the number of for-profit plans actually occurred in the mid 1980s, when the percentage of managed care providers that were for profit soared from 17 percent to 67 percent (Davis, Collins, and Morris, 1994, p. 181). Since that time, there has been no perceptible change in percentages of MCOs (69 percent) that are for-profit (Group Health Association of America, 1995a).

But market share numbers reveal another story. Between year-end 1990 and year-end 1994, the percent of HMO enrollees in for-profit managed care plans increased from 47 percent to 58 percent (Group Health Association of America, 1992, 1995b), with one organization, Kaiser, holding close to 25 percent of the nonprofit market share). And in 1994, the rate of enrollment growth in for-profit organizations (19 percent) was more than three times the 5.8 percent rate achieved by nonprofit organizations (Group Health Association of America, 1995a). Table 4.1 lists 1994 membership and market share totals for the nation's ten largest HMOs.

There is, moreover, widespread expectation that the near future may witness a significant increase in these trends, an anticipation driven in large part by expectations of conversions in Blue Cross/Blue Shield plans. In what was widely reported as a signifi-

**Table 4.1. Rise of the For-Profit HMO:
Ten Top Companies as of December 31, 1994.**

Company	Membership	Percentage of National Enrollment	For-profit/ Nonprofit Status
Kaiser Foundation Health Plans	6,599,043	12.90	Non
CIGNA HealthCare	3,309,335	6.50	For
United HealthCare	2,751,137	5.40	For
Prudential HealthCare	2,076,734	4.10	For
U.S. Healthcare[1]	1,768,094	3.50	For
FHP, Inc.	1,718,854	3.40	For
Humana Inc.	1,589,760	3.10	For
PacifiCare Health Systems	1,417,018	2.80	For
Health Systems International	1,339,253	2.60	For
Aetna Health Plans[1]	1,103,585	2.20	For

Source: Adapted from Group Health Association of America, 1995a.

[1] Aetna to acquire U.S. Healthcare in 1996.

cant change in long-standing policy, the National BC/BS association decided in 1994 to permit the use of the Blue Cross/Blue Shield name in a for-profit context. As of March 1995, three Blues plans had spun off for-profit subsidiaries, the most prominent of which was Wellpoint Network in California. At least some others are expected to follow suit (Tokarski, 1995).

Overall, as one researcher—Glenn Melmick of UCLA—estimated, as many as two-thirds of the nation's nonprofit MCOs may convert to for-profit status or sell to investor-owned chains (Rundle, 1995a).

The Rise of National MCOs

Moving in concert with the for-profit trend, is a trend toward national (including commercial insurer as opposed to local and independent) managed care companies. Between 1988 and 1994, the percentages of HMO enrollees in plans owned by national chains or commercial insurers increased from 39.5 percent to 53.5 percent, and to 60 percent by some accounts ("The Race to Consolidate," 1995), while those enrolled in independent organizations (mostly smaller, regional HMOs) declined from 32 to 21 percent[2] (GHAA, representative, interview, 1995). Table 4.2 outlines these and related trends.

Reasons for Consolidation Among MCOs

Some analysts, consumers, and others are disturbed by such trends. But there is not much controversy concerning the reasons behind them. MCOs are attempting to strengthen their competitive hand, primarily in terms of expanding market share and power. In many respects, these efforts are not much different from those of hospitals and physicians.

Clearly, some economies of scale are involved, especially in spreading the high cost of new information technologies and systems across a larger enrollment base. Reducing the unit costs of such services can assist MCOs in securing themselves in the contractor role. It can also enable them to market those services to others.

Economies of scale may also be particularly relevant in understanding the acquisition of smaller by larger HMOs. Research suggests that the greatest potential to achieve economies of scale may be in smaller HMOs, with 100,000 enrollees. Above this size additional economies of scale may be modest, which suggests both that smaller organizations may face increasing market liabilities, and that they may be ripe for acquisition by larger organizations. Given that 75 percent of HMOs have enrollments below this level (Anders and Winslow, 1995), most analysts presume there may be many targets for acquisition by larger plans.

And while some find imperatives and opportunities in growth, others find those opportunities constrained, especially by restricted access to another key strategic asset, capital. Particularly weak in this regard may be provider-owned plans. For example, MD Health

---

[2]These figures, as well as those in the list of percentages, are offered with some caution. Definitions of different forms of ownership status can change.

Table 4.2. Percent Enrollees in HMOs, by Ownership of HMO.

	1988	1994
National Chains	29.3	39.2
Commercial Insurers	10.2	14.3
Blue Cross/Blue Shield	14.9	14.9
Provider-owned	7.3	7.4
Independent	32.0	20.7
Other	3.8	3.6

Data given to author by Group Health Association of America in 1995.

Plan of Connecticut was a prototype for health plans organized by medical societies and achieved considerable success in its market. But largely due to a lack of capital, it had limited capacity for growth. It was purchased by Health Systems International for $100 million in 1995, paying considerable profit to member physicians.

Mergers and acquisitions among MCOs may be particularly likely where they serve the strategic objectives of providing easy access to new regional or product markets, and offering the broader geographic coverage and one-stop shopping required to service large employer contracts. Thus the acquisition of MetraHealth by United HealthCare brought together an HMO (UHC) specializing in HMO products with one specializing in traditional indemnity plans. And Humana's acquisition of Empheses bought it a company with half its members in markets—including Dallas, Houston, and Atlanta—where Humana wished to expand. Empheses had also made greater efforts to penetrate the small-group market, one which, as has been noted, maintains considerable potential for managed care growth ("The Race to Consolidate," 1995).

Above all, though, MCO mergers and expansions are about directly increasing market share (in health care vernacular, *covered lives*) and power. Mergers or acquisitions may be the easiest means (far easier than purchasing physicians' practices or constructing new networks) of expanding numbers of covered lives. Thus, they are also the easiest means of increasing leverage over suppliers, and, most particularly, over hospitals and physicians whose revenues depend on access to those covered lives. Greater market share—in the ideal world, dominant market share—means lower provider prices, especially for the organizations contracting with rather than owning those providers.

Mergers and acquisitions are also the fastest means of increasing revenues and thus acquiring the capital to expand operations. As the capacity to further reduce costs declines and as premiums decline with competition, revenue and profit growth must come from increased enrollment. Increasing revenues (even if not profits) may also raise growth potential, attracting investors and capital. Such a desire to increase revenues may explain, for one thing, the willingness of some HMOs to compete for Medicaid contracts, the short-term profitability of which they may view as uncertain.

The Logic of the For-Profit

As for the for-profit versus nonprofit issue, requirements in the race to expand may offer advantages to the investor-owned plan. This is not just a matter of merger and acquisition capital, of acquiring other organizations or physician practices. It is also a matter of having the financial strength to withstand aggressive competition for market share in maturing markets, and of investing in information and management systems. Reports of significant losses by major business entities attempting to enter or expand market share in maturing markets are not uncommon. Indeed, some of the largest actors may be experiencing some of the largest losses. Presumably, these organizations—particularly some of the best–known commercial insurers—believe that once a level of market share and power are established, profits will return.

But with a few exceptions, nonprofits tend to be smaller players. Many may not have the resources to wait. If content, as many may be, to simply maintain market share where they have a well-established presence, independents and most nonprofits may find the lack of access to capital markets only a modest liability. But those seeking expansion to new markets may find the more limited options of the nonprofit a much more serious liability.

Increases in numbers of IPAs and PPOs relative to staff and group model HMOs may also fuel the for-profit trend. Because they do not provide services directly, IPAs are not likely to qualify for tax-exempt status. Nor, as commercial insurers, are PPOs. Thus, the types of managed care forms that are growing the fastest may require the companies offering them to be for-profit. The same may prove true for plans offering POS benefits, which may be judged—depending on the extent of out-of-network usage—to be commercial insurance (Boisture, 1994).

Consolidation in the Hospital Industry

At some point during 1994 or 1995, just about every hospital or physician trade journal ran at least one article (often a whole magazine) on "merger mania" in the hospital sector. Whether anecdotal or systemic in nature, these articles documented a dramatic increase in merger and acquisition activity, including the strengthening of hospital chains and systems. Clearly, hospitals were responding to the new market pressures by joining forces with their own kind.

Just what "merger mania" meant, however, was a bit less clear. Unlike mergers of MCOs, in which one participant might truly disappear, merging hospitals is another story. In fact, many hospitals were reportedly finding that choosing merger partners was, relatively speaking, the easiest part of the merger process. Finalizing the merger was far more difficult; actually merging systems—especially clinical systems and departments, and perhaps closing a hospital—was even harder. As one insider commented, "Right now they are all choosing partners; dancing is another thing."

Overall, hospital consolidation activity may be both more and less than meets the eye. On the one hand, potential activity is everywhere, reflected in the myriad of ill-defined terms employed to describe the varieties of relationships contemplated and undertaken—alliances, strategic partnerships, affiliations, cooperative ventures, networks, and so on. On the other hand, most partners find conceptualization easier than implementation. What is planned may never happen; and if it does, it may not do or mean all that was intended.

The Extent of Merger Activity

For our purposes here, the wave of consolidation might be perceived as encompassing three elements: hospital mergers, acquisitions, and joint ventures; the increasing size and visibility of hospital chains, especially on the for-profit side; and, somewhat less tangible, the emergence and increasing prominence of regional hospital systems.

On paper at least, the sudden increase in 1994 merger and acquisition activity is truly striking—with hospitals merging, hospital chains purchasing more hospitals, and chains acquiring chains. Between 1980 and 1991, the American Hospital Association reported 195 mergers or acquisitions, involving just over 400 hospitals. During 1992 and 1993 there were only 32 such transactions (Health Information Resources Group, 1994). In 1994 alone, however, there were reportedly 176 mergers involving just over 300 hospitals,[3] and if acquisitions of chains by other chains are included, approximately 10 percent of the nation's 6,000+ hospitals may have been involved in merger or acquisition activity in 1994 alone.

In some cases, a market-by-market analysis could report even more striking numbers. In Massachusetts, for example, the number of hospitals declined from 141 to 91 between 1967 and 1995. In 1995 alone, twenty-six hospitals were involved in mergers (including the prestigious Massachusetts General and the Brigham and Women's Hospital) or corporate affiliations with other hospitals or managed care plans; another 6 hospitals were acquired by another hospital; and 20 hospitals entered contractual affiliations with another hospital (Zeckhauser, 1995). All told, 70 hospitals were involved in significant consolidation activity.

The For-Profit Chains

The most dramatic, and certainly the most widely heralded, of consolidation activity was among for-profit hospital chains, especially the chain of Columbia/HCA. In 1994 and 1995, about 375 investor-owned hospitals were acquired by another investor-owned chain. Most of these involved Columbia, which owned 95 hospitals at the outset of 1994, some recently acquired from the Galen chain. Columbia then added 97 more in a $5.7 billion stock transaction with the Hospital Corporation of America. In 1995, Columbia

---

[3]Numbers of such mergers can vary. Some surveys include mergers in the process, but not yet finalized. Other differences in the definition of *merger* also complicate analysis.

arranged to add another 116 by acquiring still another investor-owned chain, HealthTrust. And, as if that wasn't enough to make Columbia's CEO Rick Scott the talk of every health care conference, Columbia/HCA announced literally dozens more mergers, acquisitions, or joint ventures in 1994 and 1995, including some with academic health centers and Catholic hospitals. Such efforts appeared to clearly signal that the nation's leading for-profit chain was now looking at the nonprofit market (Lutz, 1994).

When the purchase of American Medical International by National Medical Enterprises (two other investor-owned chains), is added to Columbia's acquisitions, approximately 50 percent of all for-profit hospitals (and a larger percentage of for-profit beds) are now owned by two for-profit chains. (Estimate includes data from Shactman and Altman, 1995, and Luke, interview, 1995).

For-Profit and Nonprofit Hospitals

The highly visible market activity of the for-profit hospital chains has led many to assume that the rise of the for-profit hospital (like the rise of the for-profit MCO) and the reduction of the traditional nonprofit dominance of the hospital sector are inevitable trends.

But, at least for the time being, such a prediction appears premature. While Columbia/HCA has moved to purchase some nonprofits, to date the vast majority of its expansion has been in the acquisition of other for-profit chains. The proportion of hospitals that remain nonprofit is still well over 80 percent; 56 percent of hospitals (65 percent of beds) are owned by nonprofit corporations while 31 percent (25 percent of beds) are owned by government (Boisture, 1994). Moreover, large numbers of nonprofits remain highly profitable, and many reportedly maintain substantial cash reserves.

And while many view Columbia's Scott as the most savvy of hospital entrepreneurs—invoking both acquisition and downsizing strategies simultaneously—many wonder about the long-term prospects of Columbia's rapid expansion. Specifically, they question the value of enormous investment in a sector now riddled with overcapacity.

Still, if the numbers of for-profit hospitals may not be increasing as dramatically as is sometimes assumed, their influence may be another matter. Here a number of considerations appear relevant. For one thing, in a time when capital needs—for acquisitions of physician practices and hospitals and establishment of information systems—may be paramount, for-profits may be advantaged.

Additionally, recent trends in revenues and profit suggest that for-profit hospital profits are rising while those of nonprofits are shrinking, resulting in operating profit margins that were twice as high for for-profits (10.5 percent) as for nonprofits (4.3 percent) (Greene and Lutz, 1994). Such numbers may suggest that for-profits are more capable of rapid adjustment to fast-changing markets. For example, as many suggest is the modus operandi of Columbia, for-profits may be more willing to consolidate or even close services and facilities, reduce staffing, and take greater advantage of economies of scale. In the process, they may become more efficient, leading to gains in market share, and ultimately market power.

Finally, for-profits heading up systems that involve both for- and nonprofits may find leadership in those systems easier to come by. Joint ventures with nonprofits may leave the nonprofit as a separate entity, with its own board. But with the for-profit chain producing most if not all the capital for the joint venture, one wonders if corresponding influence in the joint venture and ultimately over the nonprofit is far behind.

Joint Ventures Between For-Profit and Nonprofit Hospitals

Columbia/HCA's joint venture approach may complicate the debate over for-profit and nonprofit hospital leadership. In these efforts, including one with Tulane's nonprofit University Hospital, Columbia/HCA spearheads a joint venture comprised of for-profit hospitals it owns and one or more nonprofit hospitals. Under the arrangement, the nonprofit hospitals are likely to keep their names, their community boards, and, presumably, their commitment to charitable care. Both parties contribute assets; the nonprofits contribute operating assets, Columbia may contribute hospitals it owns and cash.

Under such an arrangement, Columbia/HCA provides capital to the venture, but does not have to fund the purchase price of the entire hospital. If all goes well, economies of scale and efficiencies in delivery of care are achieved. Cash may be available to provide new information systems. The degree of power held by different governing boards on the board of the new joint venture may vary.

Columbia assumes the role of managing partner, responsible to the board of the joint venture. To enhance their level of commitment, physicians may be allowed to obtain equity in the new venture.

Obviously, both parties may stand to gain in such an arrangement. Public interest might conceivably be served as well, as nonprofits (which might otherwise have found it necessary to convert) maintain their nonprofit status and their commitment to charity care. But it isn't hard to see why the arrangement may raise concerns to those worried about the rise of for-profits and the fate of systems they may influence (Cain Brothers, 1995).

The Hospital System

As important as the rise of mergers and of the for-profit chains may be, the most significant of the trends in hospital consolidation may be the rise of regional hospital systems. Defined a wide variety of ways—by joint ownership, leasing, or management, or by strategic partnerships—hospital systems are, according to many analysts, growing more prominent and more dominant. While different surveys and researchers may apply different definitions, approximately 50 percent to 60 percent of community hospitals were in a system of some kind by 1994 (Greene and Lutz, 1994). By one calculation, the numbers of acute care hospitals in systems rose by 14 percent between 1989 and 1994. In metropolitan areas of over 450,000 population, fully two-thirds of all general acute care, nonfederal hospitals were involved in systems (Luke and Olden, 1995). Figure 4.1 details the distribution of hospital systems in various markets.

There may still be no widely accepted means to categorize such systems. They may vary, for one thing, by leadership, which may be provided by for-profit chains like Columbia/HCA (which generally tends to own several hospitals in a market), by academic health centers (most notably in New York City and to a lesser extent in Chicago), by church-based institutions, or by other prominent regional hospitals.

Hospital systems will also vary by scope of activity and degree of collaboration. Participation may entail modest-scale joint ventures such as building a community clinic or making joint pur-

Figure 4.1. Rise of the Hospital System: Percent of Hospitals in Systems or Networks, by Metropolitan Statistical Area.

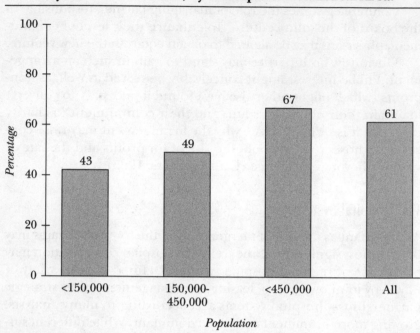

Source: Luke and Olden, 1995.

chases of equipment, or a variety of other activities well short of full merger. For a multitude of reasons including the need to maintain separate boards or to avoid antitrust scrutiny, or to avoid conflict resulting from clashes in culture, definitions of community needs, or differing religious affiliations, many hospitals find some form of collaboration or joint venture much easier to achieve than full merger.

At the other end of the scope-of-activity or collaboration continuum, hospital system activity can entail the formation of hospital-based ODSs—including vertical relationships with physicians. The merger of EHS Health Care and the Lutheran General Healthsystem in Chicago, or the merger of the Massachusetts General Hospital and the Brigham and Women's Hospital in Boston, are but two of many examples of such major health system endeavors.

But whatever the definitions applied, leadership modes, scope of activity, level of collaboration, and so on, what is becoming clear is that increasing numbers of regions may soon be defined by the existence of a small number of such systems. And, most significantly, this may be especially true where managed care penetration is higher, suggesting a clear linkage between the rise of managed care and resultant perceived need of hospitals to collaborate and consolidate.

Extensive market-focused research undertaken by Roice Luke, for example, and echoed by many other observers, anticipates that in the vast majority of metropolitan statistical areas (MSAs) of 450,000 or more residents there will be no more than three or four hospital-based delivery systems. In Chicago, 50 percent of the area hospitals are now in just five systems: one headed by Columbia/HCA; one headed by a local church-based organization; two dominated by major tertiary centers; and one that is a loose alliance of some Catholic hospitals (Luke and Olden, 1995). All of Albuquerque's eight hospitals are now reported to be in one of four systems ("Friendly Hills Sold . . . ," 1994). Many major metropolitan areas, including Cincinnati, Kansas City, Minneapolis, and Orlando, are listed as having just three major systems. (The box provides more detail on the situation in Minneapolis.) And other still sizable markets, including for example, Oklahoma City and Richmond, Virginia, may have just two such systems.

It should be hardly surprising then, that many believe the days of the stand-alone hospital, like those of the solo practitioner, are numbered. Indeed, a 1994 Deloitte and Touche survey of 1,191 hospital CEOs found that 81 percent said their hospitals would not be stand-alone facilities in the year 2000. And more than half the respondents anticipated that within five years they would be part of an integrated system (Shriver, 1994).

Reasons for Consolidation in the Hospital Sector

Like the consolidation engulfing MCOs, consolidation in the hospital sector clearly reflects the strategies outlined earlier aimed at assuring survival if not leadership in the new managed care marketplace. And, as was the case with consolidation among MCOs, the drive for market share and power are predominant here.

Hospital Consolidation in Minnesota

When it comes to consolidation, Minneapolis/St. Paul is without question the national front-runner. Largely as a result of large-employer pressure on the state's HMOs, the new paradigm of hospitals as cost centers rather than revenue centers took hold more quickly and more firmly than in other markets. Between 1982 and 1993, six hospitals closed, reducing the number of beds by almost 30 percent. By the end of 1992, of the nineteen area hospitals, all but five were in one of three hospital systems (Governance Committee, 1993).

Economies of Scale

Surely, there are some economies of scale to be achieved, and certainly all are interested in lowering system costs. Indeed, it is striking that in a era of rapidly declining utilization, and with hospitals functioning at about 63 percent of capacity, 75 percent of hospitals are still profitable (Slomski, 1995). Such continuing profitability results, in part, from aggressive cost-cutting efforts. Continuing hospital profitability may also result from the strategy of expanding services and increasing revenues from other ventures such as outpatient services, imaging centers, and home-health agencies.

But, with the possible exception of some for-profits, it is far from clear that the merger and acquisition activity so prominent among hospitals today is yielding very much in the way of economies of scale or efficiencies. Most reports suggest that savings from merger-related activities are in the 8 percent to 12 percent range. And even these savings are largely dependent on sizable infusions of capital for information systems and on the ability to consolidate sites (for example, two cardiology departments become one, and in one place) the latter of which is widely acknowledged to be the most difficult to achieve of all merger goals. Moreover, even site consolidation may not produce savings if the consolidation results in a loss of patient volume. In other words, the merged hospitals need to be in control of the contracts, thus maintaining the capacity to direct patients to one hospital or the other (Thornburg, 1995; see also Health Care Advisory Board, 1994).

In short, consolidation efforts may produce less—in terms of short-term savings at least—than is often anticipated. As merger consultants note, problems of all kinds abound. Consider, as one consultant noted, the difficulties of merging hospital salary scales when one hospital workforce is unionized while the other is not.

Market Share and Power

If consolidation may yield limited economies of scale, the relationships between consolidation and market power and share may be another matter. Controlling a sizable share of the market—be it through merger or system activity—can increase leverage over physicians, and even more important, over MCOs. Increasing leverage over MCOs in particular will, in turn, enhance the hospital's capacity to raise prices or reject demands for discounts. As a result, it is the potential for hospital mergers to generate excessive market share and power that makes them, as compared with mergers of MCOs, a key target of antitrust enforcement. As we shall see in Chapter Seven, the ability of new players to enter markets is considered critical to keeping markets competitive. New entry is much easier for MCOs, requiring the establishment of a provider network and access to purchasers. New entry for a hospital competitor involves construction or purchase of multimillion dollar facilities.

Merged hospitals and hospital systems that are able to secure relationships with primary care physicians may find their market power particularly enhanced, especially in negotiations with MCOs. Which explains, in large part, why hospitals are so intent on securing such relationships. Affiliation with a major tertiary or prestigious academic center—even if higher cost—may also increase market power, especially if the numbers of such centers in a region is limited.

But mergers or acquisitions involving major tertiary or academic centers may have particularly unique purposes, including the establishment of a core hospital around which to construct an ODS. From the point of view of the tertiary or academic center, involvement in or development of a hospital network can provide sources of referrals while meeting other needs as well. Thus, the UCLA Medical Center proposes to merge with the smaller Santa Monica Hospital, which specializes in primary care and maternity services, and which can also serve as a training center for the primary care physicians UCLA intends to recruit into a larger network. UCLA envisions its hospital serving as a hub for smaller hospitals and primary care clinics throughout much of Los Angeles. The fact that the Santa Monica Hospital has been successful in attracting managed care contracts, presumably, is hardly lost on UCLA.

Hospital Systems as ODSs or HMOs

When the hospital system covers a broad enough geographic area, achieves a needed balance of tertiary and other hospital services, and, perhaps most important, secures primary care physician relationships, hospitals and hospital systems may be far down the path of achieving the critical goals outlined earlier. They can then seek to control more of the premium dollar, accepting full-risk capitated contracts from MCOs or, if allowed, directly from employers. They can begin to serve, in short, as ODSs. They may even, if they choose to, compete with MCOs by forming their own HMO.

The hospital system may not, of course, choose to take the leap into HMO status. If nothing else, doing so will put it into direct competition with the MCOs upon which it is dependent for most of its contracts. But clearly, most hospitals engaged in merger and system development anticipate seeking managed care contracts and forming, or being part of, ODSs. Thus, mergers and system development are clearly aimed at increasing access to and control over the premium dollar.

Ideally, as hospital systems form, they will reduce excess capacity, allowing—even in the face of fewer competitors—for more competitive pricing of services. In a less optimistic scenario, reductions in capacity and economies of scale will remain elusive, leaving systems with more market leverage but the public without the benefits of increased efficiency ultimately required for more competitive pricing.

Trends in Hospital Closures: The Trend That May Not Be

Such considerations, among other things, lead to a focus on hospital closures and downsizing. Predictions of hospital closures and bed reductions have been commonplace for some time. One

recent report, for example, concluded that reform-generated consolidations may result in as many as one-third of hospitals closing
(Shriver, 1994, reporting on a study issued by two health systems
and a national consulting firm). Another industry publication predicted in late 1994 that the spread of managed care could lead to
a reduction of 169,000 beds ("How Can Hospitals . . . ," 1994).

To policy analysts, at least, these predictions are hardly shocking. For some time now, the numbers and trends underlying them
have been widely discussed. Hospital admission rates and average
lengths of stay continue to fall; on any given night one-third of the
nation's hospital beds are empty. And in many communities and
hospitals, the numbers are much higher. In California, even with
some of the highest levels of managed care penetration in the
nation, hospitals function on average at 50 percent of capacity
("East Meets West," 1994).

Given these realities, it is hardly surprising that at least one consulting group has defined hospital closures as among the most
potentially profitable of hospital network strategies (Health Care
Advisory Board, 1994).

But while there may be many assumptions about the inevitability
of many hospital closures, the inevitable hasn't arrived yet. Data from
the American Hospital Association do indicate a decline in the number of hospitals during the 1980s. But that decline appears to have
come to halt in the 1990s (American Hospital Association, 1994).

Figure 4.2 traces the recent history of hospital closures.
Between 1983 and 1993 the number of community hospitals
declined from 5,783 to 5,261. However, most of that decline was in
the late 1980s. From 1986 through 1990, the data indicate that
there were 345 community hospital closures. But from 1991
through 1993, there were just 128 such closures. In 1993 alone, the
net reduction in the number of community hospitals was just 31,
less than 1 percent. In that year, the AHA reported 34 closures and
18 mergers. Meanwhile, 17 new general medical and surgical hospitals opened (Health Information Resources Group, 1994).

The same conclusion emerges from a review of trends in numbers of hospital beds. Between 1983 and 1992, the number of beds
declined significantly, from just over 1 million to 921,000. But in
1993, the reduction in the number of beds was an insignificant
2,000—about .002 percent (American Hospital Association, 1994).

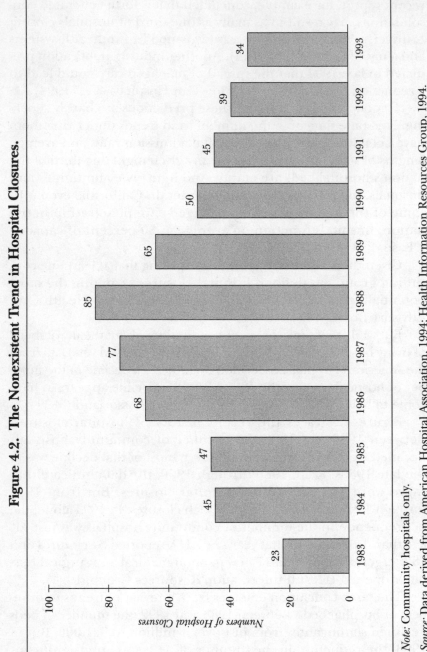

Figure 4.2. The Nonexistent Trend in Hospital Closures.

Numbers of Hospital Closures

100
80
60
40
20
0

1983 — 23
1984 — 45
1985 — 47
1986 — 68
1987 — 77
1988 — 85
1989 — 65
1990 — 50
1991 — 45
1992 — 39
1993 — 34

Note: Community hospitals only.

Source: Data derived from American Hospital Association, 1994; Health Information Resources Group, 1994.

Beds, Closures, and Politics

Such an analysis suggests that when it comes to hospital closures more may be involved than the search for efficiency, economies of scale, or even market power. The realities here may be as political as they are economic. Simply put, it can be very difficult to close a hospital. Unlike MCOs, hospitals are often centerpieces of communities. They are a major source of jobs, revenue flows, and community status. Hospital boards are often populated with a community's most prominent citizens. Indeed, one interesting preliminary finding of the ongoing Health System Change study is that employer purchasing cooperatives may be less effective and aggressive when their leaders sit on the boards of local hospitals (conference participants, 1995). Additionally, many hospitals have substantial financial reserves or independent sources of funds via trusts, as well as tax-advantaged status.

But as is the case with so many health care trends today, a few caveats must be added to such an analysis. First, hospital closures, like formal mergers, may be the third or fourth stages of consolidation efforts now in the first or second stages. Second, and again as in the case of mergers, the absence of formal closures should not imply the absence of change; many hospitals are reportedly removing capacity, or changing capacity (for example, from acute care to ambulatory or long-term care). And some analysts suggest that the expansion of for-profit hospital systems such as Columbia/HCA may facilitate or compel more hospital downsizing or closures. National for-profit systems, it is asserted, having fewer community ties or obligations and a more aggressive focus on the bottom line, may be less influenced by political or community opposition to hospital downsizing or closure.

Even the threat of such expansion may compel more aggressive hospital action. The fear of market entry by a major for-profit chain may in the view of some be enough to inspire what otherwise would not occur.

Closures and downsizing, therefore, are likely to increase over time, especially as markets mature. But for some time at least, the tension between what many believe will and must happen and what actually happens may remain.

Consolidation in the Physician Community

The emergence of managed care and its affiliated risk-sharing strategies, when combined with the impending rise of the ODS, has left some physicians with a sense of being courted—and many with a fear of being excluded. In many regions, primary care physicians are in short supply, and hospitals, MCOs, and physician management companies are bidding aggressively for their services. On the other hand, as managed care penetration increases, the oversupply of physicians, particularly specialists, grows more apparent, and fear of exclusion or removal from networks grows more intense.

Clearly, what some call the golden era of fee-for-service is dead in many communities, and probably dying in the rest. And while the new environment offers multiple opportunities for some physicians, the physician community as a whole has been slow to accept new realities. In the last few years, however, driven both by a need to defend their income and by a more aggressive desire to regain control, physicians and physician groups have been organizing and consolidating in unprecedented fashion.

The consolidation of physicians and physician practices is marked, perhaps, by three developments: first, the movement of larger numbers of physicians into group practices; second, the emergence of large medical groups—first in California, but increasingly elsewhere—as focal points of capitated managed care systems; and third, the formation of physician networks, owned and operated by physicians, that compete directly with managed care companies.

The State and Numbers of Group Practice

Many analysts believe that the formation of group practices (at least primary care, multispecialty group practices, and staff and group model HMO-type group practices)[4] is key to the expansion of organized systems and mature managed care arrangements. It is widely believed that group practices may be best equipped to

---

[4]By contrast, single specialty group practices, while capable of accepting carve-out capitation contracts, are not generally viewed as appropriate building blocks for managed care or full-risk contracts.

accept and manage capitated contracts. This would be true whether the capitation was for primary care only, for all physician services (not including hospital services), or for full-risk contracts, including all covered services.

Thus, those responsible for establishing managed care networks and systems have generally sought to build them around a group practice. Additionally, they have sought to achieve at least some level of exclusivity in the relationship between the group and the MCO, meaning that there is a core group of primary care physicians who work exclusively or almost exclusively for the MCO. Such a relationship is perceived by many to be a prerequisite for the management of capitated contracts and for achievement of a highly competitive, organized system. Where such a relationship cannot be established, looser networks of physicians under contract, including traditional IPAs, may serve as an adequate substitute. But many believe that over time such networks will not be able to compete with systems built on more integrated physician relationships.

Although it can hardly be concluded that a rise in the prevalence of group practices in the 1970s and 1980s resulted from the growth of managed care, the increase in the numbers of groups and of physicians practicing in groups between 1965 and 1991 was substantial. In that time period, the number of medical groups (including 3 or more physicians) grew by 259 percent, from just over 4,000 to over 16,000, and the number of physicians practicing in groups rose by over 600 percent, to include about one-third of nonfederal practicing physicians. Between 1988 and 1991 alone, the percentage of physicians practicing in groups rose by almost 20 percent (Havilecek, Eiler, and Neblett, 1992). Interestingly, virtually all of this increase resulted from an increase in mean group size, rather than in the number of groups. Although the latter remained essentially unchanged, the mean size increased from 6.5 to 11.5 physicians. Multispecialty groups grew from just over 11 to just over 25 physicians. The numbers of family and general practice groups grew from just under 2,300 to almost 6,000.

The great majority of groups remained small, single-specialty groups. But by 1991, multispecialty groups—while representing less than 25 percent of groups—accounted for more than 50 percent of physicians in groups. By 1991, approximately one-half of all group physicians were practicing in groups of 26 physicians or more, a size large enough to accept and manage significant levels of risk.

AMA data (as yet unpublished) for 1995 suggest at least two significant trends.[5] First, between 1991 and 1994–95 there has been a dramatic increase (20 percent) in the number of group practices—from almost 16,600 to almost 19,800. Second, there is a notable increase (26 percent) in the numbers of groups with over 100 physicians. The average size of groups remains about the same as in 1991, as does the percentage of nonfederal physicians practicing in groups (Havilecek, Eiler, and Neblett, 1996).

Anecdotal reports lend support to the new AMA data, suggesting a significant movement toward the formation of group practices. However, there may also be counterforces at work, restraining such a movement. The current success of the independent practice association model—which offers some of the benefits of a group and enables more physicians to maintain independent practices—and the efforts of medical organizations to establish networks of independent physicians may be allowing more physicians to stay in independent practice than might otherwise have been anticipated. Efforts to establish clinics without walls, and the dramatic growth in management services organizations, both of which give physicians access to varieties of management services while still maintaining some level of independence, may produce a similar effect.

Still, the movement toward group practice should continue, driven not only by the need of physicians to consolidate but also by the needs of others. Some groups are being forged by insurers trying to establish core groups in emerging markets. Others are being organized (as we shall discuss shortly) by hospitals via PHOs. And even where physicians decide to remain in independent or small practices, the communications and management services now available to them—via increasingly sophisticated IPAs, clinics without walls, management service organizations, and other larger partners—may render them part of virtual if not actual groups.

---

[5]The AMA supplied a draft executive summary of the 1995 unpublished report. There may well be other significant trends that are not reported in that summary.

Physician Integration: The California-Style Medical Group

If there is a prototype of the capitation-ready, ODS-oriented physician group, many believe it lies in California. For some time now, California's physician marketplace has been marked by the prominence of large, multisite physician groups assuming large measures of risk. Today there are probably at least fifty such groups, with at least fifty physicians each (and a number have several hundred members). Many of these—especially the older ones—derive 75 percent or more of their revenues from capitated contracts, often from as many as ten or fifteen HMOs.

Many, like the Friendly Hills HealthCare Network, are multispecialty groups; some, like the Bristol Park Medical Group in Orange County, are primary care groups that contract with specialty providers, in some cases creating long-term contractual relationships modeled on the virtual integration concept. But, whether primary care or multispecialty in structure, the capitated contracts under which they function (many have fifty thousand or more covered lives) put them at risk—either directly or through contracts—for specialty and hospital care. Many are also at risk for behavioral health and pharmaceuticals. Only a few (like the Sharp-Rees Stealy Medical Group) are affiliated with hospital systems. These, clearly, are physician-driven organizations.

These groups are distinct from group or staff model HMOs where, as in the case of the Kaiser Permanente Medical Group, high percentages of physicians are likely to work in one central location, and where the group is likely to contract exclusively with one HMO. The California groups contract with a number of HMOs. Nor do they operate like most of the nationally known multispecialty clinics—like the Mayo or Cleveland clinics. Compared to these clinics, the California medical groups are far more primary (as opposed to specialty) care-oriented, more dispersed, less hospital-based (indeed, few own hospitals), and more likely to have equity-based as opposed to salaried physician payment structures. Above all, they are far more reliant than the traditional clinics on managed care and capitated contracts, and clearly more tailored—given a primary care emphasis and geographic dispersion—to pursue and manage such contracts.

Finally, the California medical groups are also clearly distinguishable from physician-led networks in other parts of the country, many of which, as we shall see, are pursuing capitated contracts. The California groups generally achieve much higher levels of integration between physicians and the group, and invoke much stronger management styles and utilization management techniques than network-type physician efforts in other parts of the country. As a part of that management style, many have been much more aggressive about reducing the ratio of specialty to primary care physicians, often generating considerable dissatisfaction among specialty providers dropped from contracts.

Not surprisingly, as a result, the California groups are often cited (as noted earlier) for achieving lower, sometimes dramatically lower, levels of hospital utilization and specialty referral rates, and for reducing overall capitation rates. According to the Unified Medical Group Association, a trade association representing groups dedicated to managed care and capitation, their member groups (ninety in all) have average inpatient utilization rates of 150 days per thousand commercial enrollees, and 900 days per thousand Medicare enrollees, well below comparable national HMO averages (Alan Zwerner, interview, 1995). And according to recent detailed case studies of six of the California groups, commercial days per thousand for the six groups ranged from 120 to 149, with Medicare days per thousand at 643 to 936. These utilization rates are 40 percent below the California HMO average of 232 days for commercial enrollees, and 33 percent below the California HMO average (1,337 days) for Medicare enrollees (Robinson and Casalino, 1995).

These reductions, moreover, have often been achieved by primary care groups accepting full-professional-risk or full-risk contracts and contracting for specialty and hospital services. Their success in achieving such reductions has led many analysts to revisit the argument that bringing primary care physicians, specialty physicians, and hospitals into a single integrated system is the most effective strategy.

In operating as they do, the California groups also remind us of how classifications and evaluations of managed care groups can grow obsolete. As noted earlier, some would define the California groups as participating in a group model arrangement, some would define it as a network model. Where the group operates an IPA, the definitions may achieve total breakdown.

The California Experience: Unique, Benchmark, or Trend?

Many assume that the California medical group model, or at least the concept of larger and more dispersed group practices, will spread to other regions. These analysts point to the inherent strength of the model in terms both of its appeal to physicians, who maintain clinical control, and in terms of its proven capacity to function as a base for capitated ODSs. These analysts (relying largely on anecdotal data) also point particularly to the growth of larger group practices in other regions, even in the northeast, never a hotbed of group practice activity. In 1994, for example, two of New England's largest group practices agreed to merge, creating the Lahey/Hitchcock clinic, reportedly the third-largest group practice in the nation (Solovy, 1995).

The California experience, on the other hand, could remain a primarily California experience. Even with the expansion of group practices elsewhere, as many as 50 percent of groups with fifty or more physicians may operate in California. And, clearly, California groups have a unique and long history, growing up over many years in an increasingly managed care environment in which all had to compete with Kaiser.

In other regions, market transformation is occurring more rapidly, often condensing into a few years what evolved in California and Minnesota over a decade or more. Physicians elsewhere may have less time to accommodate to group practice models, with other alternatives often pressed upon them, and MCOs and hospitals sometimes having little interest in seeing physicians affiliate in large groups that might assert real market power and compete with them for leadership in organized systems.

Additionally, in other states, where both physician groups and HMOs have been less of a factor, hospital systems may be more likely to assert leadership in the development of organized systems, consolidating physicians around hospitals—often by purchasing their practices—rather than medical groups. Physicians in other regions, less accustomed to the group practice model, may also gravitate more to IPA-type models. As detailed in Chapter One,

IPAs are the fastest growing HMO type, in part due to the relative ease with which they can be organized. IPA structures can also appeal to both MCOs wishing to avoid ownership relationships with physicians and to physicians interested in maintaining higher levels of practice independence. Moreover, as also pointed out in Chapter One, some IPAs may be capable of achieving much higher levels of productivity than once assumed.

One interesting distinction that may be emerging, according to some observers, is that medical groups forming outside California are more likely to be organized and led by primary care providers. This tendency may reflect the growing awareness of primary care physicians that they have the opportunity to control more of the capitated dollar, and that most specialty services can be obtained under contract—often at considerably less cost.

Overall, then, in spite of its apparent success, it is far from obvious that the California group model will achieve dominance, or even prominence, in other markets. Thus, whether that model remains unique, a benchmark, or a trend remains a question mark.

Physician-Owned Plans and Networks

While more groups and larger groups continue to organize, many of them more capable of managing capitated contracts, some physicians and their associations are gearing up to directly compete with MCOs by establishing their own HMOs.

Such efforts can have compelling appeal to physicians, offering the potential to increase or maintain control over clinical decision making, protect themselves from exclusionary practices of MCOs, and reduce direction from distant managed care administrators. And, if they must lower prices to compete, at least they might replenish the lost revenues by capturing a share of the premium dollar now going to insurers.

Physician-owned plans, most of which are PPOs, now serve less than 10 percent of managed care plan enrollees (Group Health Association of America, 1995b). But according to recent reports, physician-led plans are likely to become a true growth industry. In New Jersey, 3,500 physicians contributed $5,000 each and raised over $17 million to establish an HMO; in New York,

MD Health Plan of Connecticut

Some physician-led HMO efforts have achieved significant success. For example, consider MD Health Plan of Connecticut, which was described briefly earlier in this chapter. Founded in 1987 and sponsored by the Connecticut medical society, the plan raised funds by requiring participating physicians to purchase shares in the organization. Established as an IPA model, and invoking withholds and risk-sharing payment methodologies, it was in the black within fifteen months of obtaining a license. However, perhaps reflecting the weakness of physician-led plans in accessing capital for expansion, the plan was sold in 1995 to Health Systems International.

the Long Island Physician Holdings Corporation is doing the same (Freudenheim, 1995b).

Additionally, about twenty state medical societies (including those in California, Florida, and Pennsylvania) are undertaking efforts to mobilize such networks (Jaklevic, 1995). To assist physicians in these endeavors, the AMA has established a program to link groups of physicians with consulting and management assistance.

To support such efforts on the political front, physicians advocate that the federal government assist physicians in starting plans by creating low-interest loan pools and providing physician networks with exemptions from various state regulations or antitrust provisions. Physicians have also been leading the fight, as we shall see later, to open up the possibilities of direct contracting between employers and providers.

The outcome of these efforts remains uncertain. But should Congress either grant physicians antitrust exemptions in organizing networks or allow physician networks to meet reduced solvency and other regulatory requirements, the physician-owned network approach would receive a sizable boost. Not surprisingly, MCOs are aggressively opposing these physician-sponsored efforts.

Even should they win long-sought exemptions, however, most analysts remain highly skeptical of physician efforts to launch and operate HMOs. Such skepticism generally stems from one or more of several assumptions.

Many medical-society-led endeavors, for one thing, may remain cautious and defensive in nature, unwilling to take the leaps necessary to compete. For example, many are unwilling to make tough choices regarding physician selection and closed panels, preferring to open the network to all member physicians. In a similar vein, most such groups continue to pay discounted fee-for-service rates, rather than capitation. Even more limiting may be the preference of such organizations for the PPO model, which offers only marginal capacity to generate reductions in utilization and costs.

Additionally, access to capital continues to be a major problem for physician-led networks. Per physician assessments can get a plan started, but capital is also required for modern management and information services, and to survive price competition struggles with better-capitalized insurers or hospital-led systems. Thus, many believe that physician-led plans will need to adopt more aggressive management styles and find allies with greater access to capital.

But many of these reservations, it should be noted, may not apply to physician-led organizational efforts based on large group practices. Especially in coalition with a larger partner with greater access to capital, these group practices clearly have capacity to operate efficient managed care plans. Indeed, many may decide to secure licenses and compete directly with MCOs.

Reasons for Consolidation in the Physician Sector

Although there is still little systematic data to demonstrate it, consolidation activity of physicians may equal that of MCOs and hospitals. In many regions, according to reports, physicians are forming more groups, expanding the size of existing groups, and increasing the levels of integration-oriented activity within groups and even within IPAs. Additionally, there are reports that multi-specialty groups are accepting and encouraging more leadership from primary care physicians.

But, in many instances, as is the case with many hospitals, physicians' and physician associations' responses to changing circumstances appear defensive. Some of their most visible efforts, in fact, have been to try to reverse rather than mould or adapt to managed care trends.

Which probably should not be surprising. Those physicians, for one thing, who might gain the most from the new environment, primary care physicians, have been generally low on the professional totem pole. Specialists have been both far more prominent in physician organizations and hospitals and far more negatively affected by the rise of managed care.

Primary care physicians, for their part, have been hit with a bewildering array of demands and opportunities. Economic realities may require them to alter their practice circumstances—moving to groups and risk-sharing strategies—and many, understandably, find the adjustment difficult. On the other hand, in many markets, MCOs, hospitals, and physician management companies are all competing for their business and loyalties.

If nothing else, physicians may be slower to adjust because they operate smaller businesses and lack access to managers, consultants, and financial planners. Additionally, it may have taken longer in many markets for physicians to understand the coming changes, or for those changes to reveal their full impact. But there is at least increasing anecdotal evidence that while some are still fighting rearguard actions, many are looking ahead and positioning themselves for new roles. As was the case with MCOs and hospitals, consolidation may be the first result.

By forming larger groups, physicians are preparing themselves to accept capitated payments, bear and manage greater amounts of risk, and position themselves and their groups to perform a central role in ODSs. Expansion of group size may also promote efficiency and economics of scale. Indeed, as groups expand they assume more of the functions of physician management, perhaps even establishing management services operations and subsidiaries.

Depending upon market size, group size, and other factors, expanding the size of group practice may also enable physicians to gain market power and share, rendering MCOs and hospitals in greater need of their services. Smaller groups may lack such leverage. Moreover, as we shall see later, short of the formation of a group practice and the sharing of risk it entails, efforts of physicians to negotiate with payers may run afoul of antitrust standards and be considered price fixing.

If physicians could secure capital and greater management and informational expertise, their leverage could be further strengthened. But securing these attributes may require partnerships with others.

Consolidation and Public Policy

Above all, the consolidation efforts of MCOs, hospitals, and physicians raise critical issues relating to antitrust enforcement and to threats to end the means of maintaining competitive markets. These are discussed in Chapter Seven.

Consolidation efforts have also raised a multiplicity of other issues, including the potential for direct contracting between employers and providers; the prospect of a significant decrease in the numbers and influence of nonprofit hospitals and the potential impact of that decrease on the ability of the overall system to deliver charitable care; the nature of the process by which nonprofit organizations convert to for-profit status; and the value or appropriateness of offering physician-led networks various forms of statutory or financial assistance. These issues will be discussed in Chapters Seven through Ten.

Matters relating to economic consolidation tend to wind up in regulatory or judicial arenas. But, it will argued later, some of the issues raised by today's consolidation of health care services need to be addressed from broader points of view than those likely to dominate regulatory or judicial proceedings. Specifically, there often is a pressing need for more focus on relationships between marketplace developments and a variety of public needs and responsibilities. In these kinds of circumstances, courts and regulators have a role, but it is to interpret and enforce—not make public policy.

Chapter Five

Next Steps
Toward Vertical Integration

Efforts to achieve vertical integration among MCOs, hospitals, and physicians have assumed myriad forms. But, to date at least, the main object of these efforts has been primary care physicians. As a result, much of the vertical integration in today's marketplace has entailed efforts on the part of those forming managed care, capitation-oriented delivery systems to secure the services and sometimes the allegiance of primary care physicians.

Efforts to secure these linkages and services involve all the major actors. Hospitals perceive their ability to form organized systems— and to secure managed care contracts and achieve market power vis a vis other hospitals and MCOs—to be dependent on their ability to generate and support an affiliated physician organization that can manage care and generate referrals. Indeed, once having done so, they can—as can other provider-driven organizations— contemplate another step in vertical integration, namely the formation of their own MCO.

MCOs—at least those wishing to direct delivery systems themselves—also find themselves needing to secure primary care relationships. With hospitals and physician management companies undertaking efforts to control physician groups and networks, and with more physician-led networks organizing, managed care companies may now find that securing ties with primary care physicians is a more competitive enterprise.

Physician management companies that manage and sometimes own parts or all of physician practices, groups, and networks are also vying for primary care physician ties. Thus, in addition to their efforts to improve management efficiency, the companies that wish to provide full service will own or manage networks, market them to MCOs, run IPAs, or even assume the role of insurer. But whatever their modus operandi, their focus is primarily on the physician group.

Obviously, the requirements of hospitals, MCOs, and physician management companies offer physicians a variety of vertical integration options. These are particularly available to primary care physicians. (Options of specialists may be far more limited.) And, like hospitals, physicians may pursue vertical integration by forming and marketing their own managed care entity. As discussed in Chapter Four, such an endeavor may require participation of partners with more access to capital than may be available to physicians acting on their own.

In this chapter, we examine linkages among MCOs, hospitals, and physicians, with special focus on linkages involving primary care physicians. We shall first review hospital-led efforts to establish physician ties through PHOs. We turn then to efforts by MCOs and hospitals to purchase practices from, employ, contract with, and otherwise cement ties with primary care physicians. Finally, we shall examine the new and expanding organizational role played by the physician management company.

New Partnerships: Physicians and Hospitals

PHOs come in a multiplicity of forms. Generally speaking, they are joint business ventures, usually spearheaded by hospitals, between physicians (as individuals or as a group) and a hospital. The PHO, often established as a management services organization with a board consisting of both physician and hospital representatives, may serve as contractor for both parties as well as management company for the physician practices, performing such functions as billing and development of information services.

Under such an arrangement, physicians can maintain considerable autonomy in their own practices, while beginning to explore managed care and other contractual relationships with a larger corporate partner.

PHOs: Numbers and Goals

By the numbers, at least, PHOs are fast becoming a major and widespread form of health system organization. Estimates of their numbers range well above 1,500, and in at least one survey, over 85 percent of hospitals reported they had established one, or intended to do so (Physician Payment Review Commission, 1995). However, while there is little doubt regarding their increasing prominence, there is considerable skepticism regarding their purposes, values, and prospects.

Some of that debate emanates from the reality that PHOs are a very recent phenomenon. The great majority—three-quarters—have been in existence less than two and a half years (Ernst & Young, 1995). But much skepticism and debate flows from an analysis of PHO goals, and whether or not those goals are achievable. As described by PHOs themselves, those goals include:

- Contracting with MCOs
- Collaborating with hospital medical staff
- Improving relationships with community physicians
- Sharing financial risk among provider participants
- Enhancing quality of care

Many observers, however, define the goals of PHOs more bluntly, citing their primary purpose as enhancing the hospitals' capacity to compete in the new managed care marketplace, and preparing to do so, in large part, by transforming the loose ties between staff physicians and the hospital into firmer relationships. The ties cemented by a PHO could provide hospitals with more leverage in negotiating with MCOs as well as greater hospital access to, if not control over, expanding outpatient revenues. In some cases, successful formation of a PHO could lead to direct contracting with employers, to the formation of a super-PHO or hospital-based HMO, and thus to direct competition with MCOs.

Limitations of PHOs

The current view among many analysts, however, is that most PHOs face major obstacles in achieving their goals, however defined. At best, they are often viewed as way stations on the road to other and higher levels of integration.

At least in terms of achieving an integrated arrangement and competing for managed care contracts, a number of problems stand out. A study undertaken by the consulting firm of Ernst and Young (probably the most in-depth survey of PHOs to date) found, for one thing, that most PHOs are specialty dominated. Whereas HMOs today may aim for a mix of 50 percent specialists and 50 percent primary care physicians, 60 percent of PHOs report that primary care physicians totaled no more than 35 percent of their membership—and fully 79 percent were under the 50 percent target (Ernst & Young, 1995). Given that specialists may have closer affiliations with hospitals than primary care physicians and may also feel more threatened in the changing marketplace, the dominance of most PHOs by specialists is not surprising. But specialists—many of whom rightly fear income reductions of 25 percent or more—may be more prone to defensive thinking, and are not likely to serve as ideal bases for organized systems or managed care contracts in which the prominence and compensation of others needs to be elevated.

Even more limiting may be the nature of PHO physician panels. Fifty percent, according to the survey, were closed panels, a network form in which the number of physician participants, especially specialists, is limited so as to direct more patient volume to network participants. However, the Ernst and Young study found that—aside from the reality that 50 percent of PHOs had open panels—the closed-panel PHOs were generally those with higher percentages of specialists (Ernst & Young, 1995). Such findings might reflect several limitations of PHOs, at least in their present form. First, they may be organized less for the purpose of forming managed care networks capable of increasing efficiency and reducing utilization, and more for the purpose of generating hospital referrals. Second, as already noted, PHOs may be dominated by specialists. And third, the process of PHO formation may reflect long-standing tensions between hospitals and physicians. Organizers may perceive a need to move cautiously, acknowledging that parties must first come to the table before they organize.

Given their limitations in organization form, it is not surprising that most PHOs have produced little evidence of increasing levels of clinical integration. Most reimburse physicians by discounted fee-for-service and report devoting few resources to systemwide integration (Ernst & Young, 1995). Many, thus, have not proceeded far beyond establishing the rubric of an organization. While some report progress in achieving financial or administrative integration, the achievement of significant clinical integration remains rare.

PHOs also face significant legal obstacles in attempting to encourage physician participation. Physicians considering PHO involvement may seek assurances that the organization will not be hospital-dominated. But funding for the PHO is likely to be supplied by hospitals, and fraud and abuse rules (dealing with kickbacks for referrals) can restrict the ability of hospitals to offer physicians more control than their financial contribution warrants. Thus, a hospital that gives physicians 50 percent control over the new PHO while contributing 75 percent of the funding may be risking a charge of paying for referrals.

Finally, many PHOs may discover that MCOs have little incentive to see PHOs thrive. Indeed, MCOs intent on organizing their own systems may compete with hospitals for the allegiance of primary care physicians. As a result, they are unlikely to have much interest in seeing those physicians linked with hospitals and achieving higher levels of market power, which would be invoked in contractual negotiations with them. MCOs, undoubtedly, also recognize that the truly successful PHO, especially a super-PHO entailing linkages of several hospitals and large numbers of affiliated physicians, may view the value-added of MCOs as a fast diminishing commodity. From there, it may be a short vertical step to an HMO license and direct competition.

Here it seems appropriate to note a critical distinction between the way MCOs may view competition with physician-led as opposed to hospital-led organizations. The former may lack capital, management expertise, sophisticated information systems, and the capacity to approach and contract with employers, all things the MCO can supply. Indeed, as already noted, many MCOs are envisioning roles in which they provide such services while turning over the actual delivery of care—and the risk associated with it—to physician-led delivery systems.

But hospital-led systems may be more capable of producing internally the services physician-led systems may have to secure elsewhere. Thus, regardless of which leadership group—physicians or hospitals—may produce the greatest value, the MCO may see a more productive economic partnership in the one rather than the other.

It may not be surprising, then, that many PHOs have experienced difficulty in securing managed care contracts and covered lives. In one instance, ChoiceCare (Ohio's largest HMO) has determined it will no longer contract with PHOs for physician services, or with physicians whose practices are owned or controlled by a hospital. The company's public rationale for this policy is its desire to promote a physician-centered rather than a hospital-centered system. But other commentators viewed the decision as reflecting a need to protect and maintain HMO leverage with providers (Sardinha, 1995b).

This reasoning, in turn, may explain the interest of many PHOs and other provider-driven systems in direct contracting with employers. If access to larger percentages of the premium dollar cannot be achieved through MCOs, perhaps it can be achieved in other ways, with either the providers or the employer assuming the functions once assumed by the insurer.

PHOs in Transition

All these limitations notwithstanding, some hold out positive prospects for at least some PHOs, at least as a transition mechanism—for both hospitals and physicians—to more fully integrated systems. From this point of view, the PHOs' greatest contribution—whatever their specific arrangements or accomplishments—may be to heighten physician awareness of the need to establish new partnerships in preparation for managed care contracting, and especially for the assumption of full-risk contracts.

As such, initial PHO efforts may serve as first steps toward larger organizational efforts, including establishment of hospital medical staffs as multispecialty groups; increased use of management service organizations aimed, among other things, at improving efficiency in physician management and coordination of contractual efforts; and, as noted earlier, creation of super-PHOs and hospital-based systems capable of accepting and competing for full-risk managed care contracts.

Moreover, data from the Ernst and Young study do suggest that, over time, more PHOs may achieve progress in managed care technique and contracting. Older PHOs have had more success in gaining covered lives. The PHO associated with Lutheran General Healthsystem in Chicago, for example, (now itself part of a larger hospital system) contracts with HMOs, including Humana, and accepts virtually full physician and hospital risk, purchasing its own reinsurance as part of the arrangement (Kertesz and Wojcik, 1994). And in Denver, a number of PHOs have abandoned open arrangements whereby they accepted all physicians and functioned primarily as marketing agents, and have become closed-panel organizations accepting full-risk contracts ("The Dynamics of Market Reform," 1994).

PHOs with more capitated contracts, like the one established at Lutheran General, also appear more likely to invoke more aggressive utilization management strategies, including more use of primary care managers and of catastrophic case management. (Significantly, however, even the more sophisticated PHOs do not, according to the survey, approach efficient HMOs when it comes to information systems and ability to track utilization patterns) (Ernst & Young, 1995).

PHOs with higher numbers of covered lives also appear more organizationally aggressive: they were, among other things, more likely (49 percent) to be anticipating a merger with another organization, and more likely (43 percent) to be giving consideration to integrating delivery and insurance functions by obtaining an HMO license.

There are, then, some grounds to conclude that PHOs have potential as building blocks of ODSs. Ultimately, there remains a more fundamental question of the capacity of hospitals to accept the new paradigm in which reducing the hospital's role is a crucial element. Some, undoubtedly, will prove capable of doing so. But the extent to which most hospital-based organizations will prove effective in spearheading such efforts remains an open question.

New Partnerships: Cementing Ties to Primary Care Physicians

Like hospitals, MCOs are pursuing a variety of new partnering relationships with physicians. And as many potential ODSs endeavor to position themselves to control larger portions of the premium dollar, many MCOs perceive a new urgency to securing these relationships.

MCOs: Ceding or Controlling Care Delivery

In many respects, the rise of the ODS construct, and the concomitant mobilization of provider-based organizations, poses—almost by definition—a potential threat to insurer-led efforts. Just as hospitals face difficult new paradigm considerations, so too do MCOs. Ever larger organizations of physicians and hospitals, often endowed with capital resources, are or will soon be capable of performing many functions once the exclusive domain of insurers. Some of these provider-led organizations have already formed their own HMOs and assumed the insurance function: others hope to seek full-risk capitated contracts from insurers, in which they, not the insurer, bear the risk—and in which they, not the insurer, control the management of care. Undoubtedly, as is already occurring, such organizations will demand from insurers a larger share of the premium dollar. Most specifically, they will argue that they, not the insurer, should receive that portion of the premium that went to risk-bearing costs.

In the face of these changes, some MCOs may cede the delivery of care and management of risk to delivery systems, and focus on other functions—including contracting, marketing, information services, and capital accumulation as their value added. Other MCOs, by contrast, that seek to maintain control over larger amounts of the premium dollar and manage the delivery system itself must, like hospitals, secure relationships with providers, especially primary care physicians.

Obviously, many MCOs already have such relationships. Staff and group model HMOs generally have long-term contractual or ownership relationships with physician groups. Other HMOs, in network or IPA models, may have contractual relationships with physicians who derive virtually all their patient revenues from that insurer; that is, they have exclusive or near-exclusive relationships.

Still, many MCOs may find their relationships with primary care physicians threatened by the rise of physician- and hospital-led networks. Such concerns and strategic needs have led many

MCOs into a variety of integrated relationships aimed at securing ties with those physicians. This appears to be particularly true for MCOs—most notably commercial insurers—that have moved from an indemnity to a managed care focus or that are trying to gain market share rapidly in new markets.

In doing so, they often face competition from hospitals, physician groups, and physician management organizations. Each of the options for building ties with primary care physicians discussed here, in fact, has been invoked not just by MCOs but by hospitals and physician management companies.

Purchasing of Physician Practices

One obvious means of securing long-term ties to primary care physicians is to purchase their practices or the clinics and groups in which they practice. For some years now, managed care plans, hospitals, other physician groups and physician management companies have all been active in such purchasing activity.

Among MCOs, some of the visible purchasing activity has been undertaken by major commercial insurance companies, often as a means of establishing a managed care presence in a market. Aetna and Prudential have been particularly active in this arena in, among other places, Atlanta, Chicago, Dallas/Fort Worth, Houston, and Charlotte, with one report indicating Prudential had increased enrollment in the Southeast from 450,000 to 700,000 in 1993 and 1994 (Garvin, Ruger, and Roble, 1994). Blue Cross/Blue Shield Associations have launched similar campaigns in Massachusetts and Georgia, among other regions. Cigna has also been involved in physician-practice purchasing activity.

In some markets, these and other MCOs may create mixed models, in which a core group of primary care practices are owned, with the rest of the network structured around contractual relationships. This approach may provide the insurer with a solid primary care physician base from which it can then negotiate contracts with other primary care providers, specialists, and hospitals. In a variation on this approach, MCOs may cement stronger ties with some primary care providers by signing exclusive (or near-exclusive) contracts in which they guarantee some physicians or groups a sizable patient flow—perhaps equal to 60 percent or more of the provider's revenues. Such contracts are likely to be more common in an insurer's primary markets, such as US Health-Care in Philadelphia. Where insurers have smaller market shares, such contracts may be less viable and less common.

To date, it is difficult to determine just who has been purchasing how many practices or groups. In this area of market activity, anecdote and rumor continue to rule. Some suggest that practice-purchasing activity is still increasing; others suggest it has already peaked and is being replaced by contractual and equity-based relationships; still others suggest that purchasing activity is still very aggressive, but more focused on groups than on individual practices. Obviously, any overall assessments must be made with considerable caution.

That acknowledged, it would appear that hospitals have been the most aggressive in purchasing practices, especially those of hospital staff physicians. In a bidding war, hospitals may be willing to pay the most for these practices, which represent their key referral sources. Losing them to a competitor who might demand that the physician direct patients elsewhere could be a devastating outcome for hospitals.

Physician management companies may be the next most active purchaser, especially of larger clinics and groups, and perhaps increasingly of specialty carve-out groups. Insurers and managed care companies may rank third on a list of purchasers, purchasing both individual practices and groups, especially when establishing networks in new or expanding markets. Finally, major medical groups—including large multispecialty clinics like Mayo—have employed practice-purchasing strategies, often to expand geographic coverage as required in managed care contracting.

But there are at least anecdotal indications that practice-purchasing strategies often fail to achieve objectives. For one thing, the strategy can be expensive, and particularly so when other competitors are also employing it. Anecdotes abound in which bidding wars have produced soaring values for the assets of primary care practices, with solo practices sometimes running into the hundreds of thousands of dollars. Group practices, depending on many circumstances, can entail costs of several hundred thousand dollars per physician. Purchases of major clinics—like the Friendly Hills Medical Group in Southern California—can soar into the tens of millions ($140 million in this case).

Not only can they be expensive, but such acquisition strategies can entail high risks. The ability to tie primary care physicians (as opposed to the assets of their practices) to the purchaser can be legally complicated and limited. Long-term contracts and detailed incentive arrangements may be required, for example, to ensure that the physician (as opposed to the practice) will continue to serve the insurer. If the physician were to accept contracts with other insurers, or retire, much of the value of the purchase would be lost. Some states, moreover, have laws barring insurers from enforcing noncompetition agreements on physicians, who retain the right to contract with other insurers. Productivity is also an issue, with many reports circulating of reductions in physician productivity after a practice sale.

Finally, many analysts point to the human nature factor in purchasing relationships. Physicians, it is asserted, are highly independent and cherish autonomy. As futurist Jeff Goldsmith observed in a widely cited article, "Physicians crave order but despise authority. . . . They are, in short, terrible employees" (Goldsmith, 1993a).

For all these reasons, some of those once active in purchasing practices may be less so today, perhaps replacing the strategy, or adding to it, with more emphasis on contracts or equity- or service-based relationships.

Equity- and Service-Based Relationships with Primary Care Physicians

Many MCOs—including both those that seek to lead delivery systems and those content to contract with them—as well as hospitals and physician management organizations have also undertaken efforts to cement relationships with primary care physicians by building equity-based partnerships with them. In such arrangements, integration entails a merging of financial interests and risk sharing. But unlike capitation or bonus strategies, in which physicians or groups may stand to gain based on their own performance, equity-based partnerships tie financial gain to performance of the system as a whole. Supposed advantages of such an approach include encouragement of a systemwide focus, greater capacity to attract high-quality and managed-care-oriented physicians, and enhanced capacity to get providers in less mature markets to accept the new paradigm of less utilization equaling greater profit.

Most important of all, perhaps, is the capacity of such a strategy to cement ties with primary care physicians via means that may increase rather than decrease productivity, and avoid the high cost of practice purchases. Invoking such a strategy, PacifiCare, for example, announced plans to sell stock to selected providers. And Healthsource, which provides HMO, PPO, and third-party-administrator products in many secondary markets, was founded on the assumption of provider-insurer partnerships (Hodapp and Samols, 1994).

Related to equity-sharing constructs are relationships in which MCOs, hospitals, and physician management companies develop increasingly complex physician management and information services, which they offer to participating providers. While not owning the practices or clinics, larger corporate partners can use the provision of such services (as well as infusions of capital) to tie physicians and clinics to them. Thus, Aetna created a physician management subsidiary—Aetna Professional Management Corporation—to manage its clinics and attract primary care physicians who might benefit from such services (Garvin, Ruger, and Roble, 1994, p. 4). United HealthCare, in another variant of such a strategy, increased ties with and leverage over its physicians by controlling the information management capability of its providers (Hodapp and Samols, 1994).

Such a strategy may become increasingly evident among MCOs willing to cede control over the delivery system while focusing more on providing value added—information and management services, capital, and so on—to delivery systems. Among other things, such strategies may serve to stave off competition from hospitals or physician management companies eager to offer these same services.

Physician Employment

Direct employment offers still another physician linkage strategy. In expanding its base beyond California, Kaiser Permanente, for example, has continued to recruit primary care physicians. Perhaps reflecting the increased competition for these physicians, at least in some regions, Kaiser Permanente has reportedly become more involved in graduate medical education, and made special efforts to attract female physicians with flexible schedules (Garvin, Ruger, and Roble, 1994). Aetna, invoking a partial employment-based strategy, has undertaken efforts to establish twelve to fifteen Health-Ways family medical centers in Houston, staffed by salaried primary care physicians who can serve as gatekeepers to Aetna plans ("The Dynamics of Market Reform," 1994).

Hospitals, too, may be employing more physicians, at least where not encumbered by laws barring the corporate practice of medicine. Overall, however, physician employment does not appear to be the currently preferred strategy of major system organizers, with hospitals being a possible exception. Among other things, the start-up costs of staff and group model HMOs, those more likely to employ physicians, are much greater than start-up costs for network or IPA arrangements, including those involving relationships with already established medical groups. Today, most MCOs appear to favor incentive-based and contractual relationships.

Vertical Relationships Between MCOs and Hospitals

In addition to efforts to secure ties with primary care physicians, MCOs may also seek vertical ties with hospitals and hospital systems. Again, such relationships are common in some HMO models, with the HMO owning hospitals as part of its system. But recently some MCOs have sought to approach the goal of integrated systems by acquiring or entering into longer-term relationships with hospitals or hospital systems.

PacifiCare HMO in California, for example, contracts on a long-term basis with Sharp HealthCare in San Diego for a system of hospitals and medical groups. The Foundation Health HMO contracts for hospital services with the Mercy Hospital system. Minneapolis HMO Health Partners merged with Ramsey HealthCare, a St. Paul hospital and physician group, with the latter's operating units becoming new divisions of the HMO. Independence Blue Cross, the largest insurer in southeastern Pennsylvania, merged with Graduate Health Systems, which owns seven hospitals and a major physician network.

Such major acquisitions, mergers, and long-term contracts can place MCOs in stronger positions in terms of securing roles in the organized systems many think will soon dominate the landscape.

But new partnering activity between MCOs and hospitals is hardly the most dominant feature of current realignment activities. Today, competition between the two appears to be far more common than collaboration. As we have seen, countless hospitals are engaged in efforts to organize hospital-based systems of multiple varieties, many of which envision the formation of ODSs capable of assuming some insurance functions. That is, they envision vertical integration via their assumption of roles traditionally performed by insurers.

Taking a very different point of view, most MCOs view the current high level of hospital overcapacity as a means of driving down hospital prices, thus offering opportunities to lower premiums, increase profits, or both. And as we have seen, most HMOs appear uninterested in capitating hospitals, a strategy that might enable hospitals to reap more of the gains of lowered utilization as well as increase their capacity to function as integrated (including vertically integrated) systems.

Thus, while room for cooperation exists, there are both long- and short-term reasons for most MCOs and hospitals to remain wary of each other's intentions and to maintain a vibrant competitive relationship.

Physician Management Companies: New Kid in Town

If any subject can rival the expansion of Columbia/HCA's for-profit hospital chain as a source of controversy and attention at today's gatherings of health care professionals and policy analysts, it is the new breed of physician management companies. In any open-ended interview about health care trends, they are frequently the first subject mentioned.

A host of factors has produced an almost startling growth in this industry. These include the rise in numbers of group practices and consolidation-oriented relationships among physicians and the need of physicians to reduce administrative costs in a more competitive environment. There is a widespread perception on the part of management companies (and Wall Street investors) of huge opportunity for growth in the management of practices and groups and the services they provide, calculated as a $200 billion industry. The growing complexities of today's contractual arrangements between physicians and larger corporate entities and the insecurity of many physicians in a fast-changing environment also contribute to the growth of physician management companies.

Sponsors, Purposes, and Services of Physician Management Companies

Sponsors of these entities vary. They may be established by hospitals, by MCOs, by large medical groups (to serve members and associates in IPAs), or—in their most visible form today—by investor-owned companies dedicated to physician practice management activities. Services provided may include recruiting, marketing, accounting, purchasing, information services functions, and contract negotiations, especially with managed care companies. In some cases, particularly those in which the dedicated companies are involved, services may also include the organization and management of physician networks—including the development and installation of comprehensive information and utilization management systems. In almost all cases, however, while the management services organization is likely to play a significant role in the management of care delivery, clinical decision making is clearly left to physicians—which is, of course, one of the elements of the arrangement that renders it appealing to physicians.

As for financial relationships, management companies may serve simply as managers of physician practices, jointly owned—perhaps in the legal form of a management services organization—by a hospital and the physicians. In other cases, the management company may own all or part of the physician practice or group. In the case of the more dedicated physician management companies, the company is likely to purchase all or part of the practice or group, taking a portion of revenues for management services. As part of the arrangement, physicians may receive stock in the company.

Investor-Owned Dedicated Physician Management Companies

Most important, perhaps, strategic purposes may vary by sponsor as well. Hospitals and MCOs may employ management companies in large part to create value added in their physician partnerships and thus tighten bonds between themselves and physicians.

By contrast, the dedicated management companies (as distinguished from those operated by an MCO or hospital) may offer physicians and groups of physicians a different value—an option to maintain independence from hospitals or MCOs, and to improve leverage in relationships with them. Several factors may enable them to offer this option, but none is more critical than the ability to provide capital to physician partnerships, presumably enabling them to improve efficiency—especially in information services—and, where possible, to expand, increasing economies of scale and market power.

Even the largest of multispecialty groups may have difficulty setting aside or raising capital reserves. The Kelsey-Seybold Clinic in Houston, for example, already one of the largest group practices in the Southwest with 175 physicians in 1992, required capital for new facilities and services (Goldfarb, 1993). It was soon acquired by Caremark International. Even the giant, California-based Mullikin Group (with almost 500 physician members) found eastward expansion difficult without additional access to capital. It considered going public, but instead allowed itself to be acquired by MedPartners, creating the first major consolidation among physician management companies.

In addition to the expansion of facilities and networks, capital is sorely needed for information systems. Thus, PhyCor, the largest of the management companies until the MedPartners/Mullikin acquisition, is reported to be investing $5 million annually in a common information system that will, among other things, track data on patients and outcomes, allowing for improvements in management of care and greater appeal to purchasers ("Friendly Hills Sold . . . ," 1994). Clearly, such investments go beyond the framework of practice management as narrowly defined, which suggests the broader potential role of the dedicated, investor-owned management companies.

As they supply capital, information services, practice management expertise, and network organization, and as their networks grow larger and achieve economies of scale, dedicated physician management organizations can provide increasing market leverage for physician participants. The MedPartners/Mullikin acquisition, for example, will create a company with about 800 physicians working in 123 medical centers spread over thirteen states ("Medpartners & Mullikin to Merge," 1995). The Caremark network includes over 450 physicians (55 percent primary care), and PhyCor, at the end of 1995 owned thirty clinics in seventeen states, including 1,700 physicians. PhyCor also operates IPAs in fourteen markets. Organizations and networks of this scope, geared to seeking and accepting full-risk capitated contracts, and capable where the opportunity arises of providing insurance as well as delivery system functions, clearly can become major influences in today's marketplace.

From the physician's point of view, as suggested earlier, a partnership with a physician management company may offer financial security coupled with autonomy in the delivery of care, and a capacity to remain independent of hospitals and MCOs. This, indeed, is one of the key sales pitches of the new industry. It sells services, leverage, security, and autonomy.

All of which, no doubt, explains why the new breed of physician management company is raising concerns among many executives of managed care firms and hospitals, as well as great interest on Wall Street, where such companies are widely viewed as among the most aggressive and entrepreneurial competitors in delivery system reform. Not ignored, of course, is the opportunity for profit in modernizing the management of a $200 billion/year business of physician services. Now a $2.5 billion industry, all the major management companies are publicly traded, and some of the largest (such as PhyCor, Coastal, MedPartners, and Pacific Physician Services) have been increasing revenues at over 30 percent a year.

It is hardly surprising then that the physician practice management industry continues to exhibit substantial growth. New organizations are emerging monthly and going public, with many apparently seeking to command niche markets. And, while the larger, more established companies have focused on purchasing large primary care and multispecialty practices (as well as some specialty groups), some of the most recent entries are attempting to command niche markets, organizing and managing physical therapists, orthodontists, ophthalmologists, and even veterinarians (Abelson, 1995).

However, in spite of Wall Street interest and a potential fit with perceived physician needs, the eventual significance and direction of the roles to be performed by these relatively new entities remains somewhat in the realm of speculation. Among other things, while every purchase or consolidation they undertake makes today's journal headlines, the percentage of physician practice revenues they actually control remains minimal. The largest of the for-profit companies, MedPartners/Mullikin, may have revenues of $1 billion in 1996—still less than .5 percent of the $200 billion physician services market. Taken together, the sixteen largest public physician management companies control less than 5 percent of the market ("Medpartners & Mullikin to Merge," 1995). And, while PhyCor may control the most groups at thirty, it should be remembered that there are probably over eighteen thousand groups today.

Additionally, physician management companies are not without competitors. Emerging hospital systems and managed care companies recognize both the dollars involved and—just as important to them—the opportunity that management services may provide to link groups and physicians to their enterprise. Indeed, because they have other reasons besides direct profit to offer such services, they may well be willing to offer them for less than the dedicated management companies can charge.

Finally, depending in part on the degree of consolidation that may occur among physicians, physician management companies may, like other major actors, face value-added questions from physicians, managed care companies, and employers. If ultimately perceived as adding another management and profit-taking layer onto the premium dollar, their case for expansion could fast grow more problematic.

Vertical Integration and Public Policy

The growth in new vertical partnerships among MCOs, hospitals, physicians and physician groups, and physician management services organizations both highlights and creates a series of public policy questions.

Some of these are legal in nature—including tax and other laws that define the kinds of financial relationships (including the ownership of physician practices) that may or may not be allowed.

Additionally, the rise of vertically integrated delivery systems raises questions as to whether or not state regulators, responsible for quality assurance and for guaranteeing the solvency of those accepting risk, need to focus more attention on the new types of integrated structures—few of which today undergo regulatory scrutiny. And certainly, the rise of these systems, like the rise of larger horizontally integrated systems, raises issues of the potential of the new systems to seek direct contracting opportunities—that is, between employers and providers. As interest in those opportunities rises, government may need to decide whether or not such relationships should be fostered, and should require some new measure of regulatory oversight. These issues are discussed in Chapters Seven and Nine.

Chapter Six

The Organized Delivery System

A focus on the capitated premium dollar—and especially on the need to secure access to and control over as much of it as possible—leads, almost inevitably, to the concept of the ODS. The core quality of such a system, after all, is its capacity to assume responsibility for a full continuum of medical services. In doing so, the system can both maximize the opportunity for profit (by controlling more of the premium dollar) and minimize the risks (by performing services itself) of accepting a capitated payment. If, by improving coordination and efficiency across the continuum of services, the ODS can improve its performance and value (lower cost, higher quality) relative to competitors, then the full potential of the system can be realized.

Such assumptions no longer require a leap of faith. Today there may be many unresolved questions as to how to best integrate parts of or coordinate activities of a delivery system; but there is considerable consensus that improved management and coordination of care can at minimum lower costs. And there are multiple reasons to hope, at least, that—properly implemented—they can improve quality as well.

Core Elements of the ODS

Analysts have used a variety of terms, each evoking different images, to describe the new delivery system structures. To describe the level of organization involved, some refer to *integrated* systems. But this term may imply more coordination than exists in most of the emerging organizations. On the other hand, referring to the new systems as *networks* ignores the potential and desire of organizers to achieve higher organizational levels. As a compromise, the term *organized system* may be the most neutral as well as the most comprehensive, encompassing both those entities that have moved substantially down a path toward integration and those that may have many of the parts in place, but are a long way from getting them to function as a coordinated whole.

As for the focus of the enterprise, it seems appropriate to stress delivery over insurance. While some emerging and some older systems include both insurance and delivery functions, it is appropriate to emphasize that the key new element of the emerging systems is the effort to organize the delivery of care.

But having chosen the terms, what do they mean? For our purposes here, we employ what might be labeled a working definition of an ODS, that is, one that focuses on the key goal or function that most systems are working toward. Thus an ODS is one that is structured to accept (and capable of accepting) clinical and financial responsibility for delivering at least the full continuum of care defined in the standard managed care benefits package.

Such a focus, whether based on logic or on a review of efforts being undertaken to maintain and create organized systems, suggests that these systems may be distinguished by their focus on the following goals or characteristics:

- *Some level of clinical, not just administrative or financial, coordination among providers along the full continuum of care.*

When the system's business is delivering medical care, the emphasis on clinical integration, as opposed to financial or administrative integration, may seem obvious. But it is important to emphasize that nearly all analysts of organized systems note that clinical integration is the hardest form of integration to achieve (Shortell, Gillies, and Anderson, 1994). Researchers have found that systems have had more difficulty achieving integration on such dimensions as clinical information systems, clinical outcomes monitored and disseminated, quality assurance/improvement, and physician involvement than they have had on such dimensions as financial management and planning, human resources planning, and market research (Coile, 1995). Especially when it comes to clinical integration, then, many groups claiming the ODS title today are doing so more out of expectation and hope than current reality. Many are still more involved in putting the pieces of a system together than in making them work as a coordinated unit. However, given that our working definition includes seeking as well as attaining certain goals, it covers many groups still in the early organizational stages.

Coordination of clinical care in an ODS may not mandate a full alignment of incentives among all providers, or a primary focus of all on outcomes of the system as a whole. But it may suggest that, at minimum, incentives should not conflict, and should be coordinated such that care is given by the most appropriate and cost-effective provider—whether that be a primary care physician, a specialist, a hospital, or any other provider.

The clinical coordination requirement also focuses attention on the assumption that care delivered by different providers be coordinated or managed. This, in turn, may require that some unit or individual (usually, but not necessarily, the primary care physician) be responsible for that coordination, and there be some communications system in place to facilitate such coordination and management.

* *A focus by at least some system actors, most likely primary care physicians, on performance of the system as a whole.*

Organized systems will ultimately be judged more on their overall performance—costs, service, quality—of the overall system than on the performance of their parts. In an ODS, for example, the issue is not whether primary care physicians, specialists, or hospitals individually produced lower costs for treating a defined population, it is whether or not system costs overall are lower. Thus such markers as numbers of referrals to specialists or hospital days per thousand enrollees may be helpful indicators but not the ultimate determinants of system performance.

An ODS, then, must build in, and have all units conscious of, some construct of overall system performance that encourages overall system coordination. And, given increasingly competitive markets and greater demands by employers, the goal here must be not only to improve system performance, but to demonstrate it. Such a requirement should increase the focus on overall outcomes, and, in turn, on the capacity to collect data on a wide variety of performance measures.

As noted earlier, the focus on system outcomes suggests an interesting relationship between capitation of providers and the ODS. Capitation may be critical in generating the drive toward provider and MCO consolidation and efficiency that marks much marketplace activity today. But in a competitive marketplace where systems are judged and providers are focused on overall performance (including cost), the value of and need for capitation of individual or small groups of providers may diminish considerably.

• *Achievement of some level of physician integration (commitment of physicians to the system) at least among primary care providers.*

Encouraging a focus on the system as a whole—including use of most appropriate and cost-effective providers and coordination among providers—may require a core of primary care providers that are significantly integrated into the system, that is, committed and tied to it and thus heavily invested in improving its performance. Such physician integration may be achieved (as has been discussed) by employment or equity-based relationships, by a long-term contract with a medical group, or, as in many networks and IPAs, by exclusive or near-exclusive contracts between the ODS and a core of primary care physicians.

• *A focus on primary care and prevention.*

In a managed care, and especially in a capitated environment, such a focus may be obvious. But it has challenging implications. Above all, it may require a shift of funds from inpatient to outpatient services, from hospitals to physicians, and from specialists to primary care physicians. None of these shifts come easily, and are that much less likely to be achieved in the absence of system building or of a focus on overall system performance.

• *A minimum geographic and service breadth.*

These are requirements for winning employer contracts, accepting and spreading risk, and covering the full continuum of care. But, again, what appears to be a modest requirement can, in a highly competitive marketplace, quickly become a very demanding one. Achieving service and geographic breadth may require capital both for system expansion and for the information systems necessary to coordinate a larger and more complicated system. Additionally, such a requirement may—depending on the nature of competitors—demand a certain minimum overall size, without which economies of scale and market leverage will prove elusive.

- *Development of sophisticated (and expensive) information systems.*

Without such systems in place—to track patient care, outcomes, utilization, claims, and a multiplicity of other measures and records, achieving goals of the organized system will be next to impossible. Both improving performance and demonstrating improvements will be more difficult; expanding the system (as required to compete in the marketplace) will result in lower levels of coordination; moving data from one provider or unit to another will be inefficient.

Among other things, this requirement will demand access to capital, which could, with considerable justification, be listed as a separate, core requirement of the ODS.

- *A capacity to improve and compete on quality.*

Many assume that the ultimate competition between organized systems will, at least over time, focus on quality. Many organized systems are, for their part, clearly preparing for such an eventually, and boast high quality as their calling card.

To the extent competition on quality does occur, it will put a premium on data collection and information systems, on effective prevention strategies, on physician recruitment procedures and ongoing physician education efforts, and on an ability to develop, implement, and monitor protocols and clinical guidelines.

But including quality improvement as a core systemic element implies a critical distinction: Raising quality involves much more than lowering utilization. Many systems appear to be demonstrating an ability to achieve the latter—and even the lower costs associated with it. And some managed care proponents, including employers, may be prone to equate lower utilization with higher quality. In some instances, of course, that equation is valid. But true quality improvement goes more to reductions in morbidity, improved outcomes of medical interventions, and overall health status of the population served. And while there are many circumstances in which improvements in these outcomes are associated with lower utilization or cost (as with many immunization programs), such overlap is not always the case, much as we might wish it to be so. Researchers still find that most medical interventions have value. And economists assume that in an efficient market raising quality relative to competitors will raise costs.

For these reasons, listing quality improvement as a central requirement of the ODS includes a healthy measure of futurism and optimism. In today's marketplace, price appears to be far more dominant than quality. Thus, a listing of ODS characteristics focused primarily on present-day achievements, as opposed to a mix of those achievements and future goals, might place more emphasis on requirements associated with reducing costs than on improving quality.

The Varied Forms of ODSs

Acceptance of a list of core ODS requirements may set the stage for the exploration of those systems. It may also suggest that some organizational forms may be inappropriate or insufficient to the tasks at hand. But it does not suggest a clear preference for a particular form of organized system. Nor does it suggest much certainty in predicting how various systems will perform or succeed.

Today's marketplace, if nothing else, suggests that such judgments would be premature. A great deal of (presumably) intelligently directed capital is being invested in a great many different types of systems. These systems vary according to a plethora of variables, including source of system leadership, levels of horizontal or vertical integration achieved, sources of capital, regional versus national leadership or ownership, breadth of services or products offered, and extent to which contractual or ownership relationships are employed. In sum, as many are quick to quip, "You've seen one organized delivery system, you've seen one organized delivery system." Each has assets and liabilities, backers and critics. And, in a marketplace as fluid as the current one, most will get a chance to prove their value.

Underlying the competition may be one central question. Under what circumstances or at what points along the continuum of care is more integration better? Certainly, this is a complex question involving a number of factors. But in the current evaluation and discussion of organized systems, three stand out. First, what might be the advantages and disadvantages of merging delivery and insurance functions in one organization? Second, what are the advantages and disadvantages of exclusive relationships between sets of providers and the system? Third, and probably most important, what are the advantages and disadvantages of contractual as opposed to ownership or employment relationships—both between insurers and delivery systems and within the delivery system itself? Can two or three organizations perform as productively—including the achievement of similar levels of desired integration—as one?

We will turn to a discussion of these questions later. But it may be helpful to keep them in mind as we outline several of the major types of systems now evolving, their distinguishing features, and the extent to which they may or may not meet the requirements of an ODS.

This section discusses some of those forms—mostly resulting from the partnering efforts outlined earlier. Our focus is less on their current, short-term economic potential for success, although short-term success may be a necessary condition for survival, and more on how they might achieve the requirements and goals of an organized system. Omitted from the list are organizational forms such as the group practice without walls or the single-specialty group that might form a part of an ODS but, in the view of most analysts, could not lead, organize, or form the core of such a system.

Some Less Integrated Organizations

A number of well-known organizational forms appear to fall short of meeting the criteria of an ODS. However, most of them appear to form potential stepping stones in the direction of the ODS.

PPOs

Even though many PPOs now invoke more sophisticated and aggressive utilization management strategies, few could be classified as organized systems. Discounted fee-for-service remains the dominant mode of payment; utilization review procedures are modest in scope and sophistication. Providers are not at risk, and there is often little systematic coordination of care across a continuum of services.

However, greater levels of integration may be achieved when the MCO operating the system directs a sizable patient volume to selected primary care physicians, generating higher levels of physician-system linkage. Higher levels of integration can also be achieved when an organized system, such as a multispecialty group or a group model HMO offers a PPO product serviced by physicians affiliated with its system. Such offerings are growing more common, and may blur distinctions between PPOs and other more highly controlled and coordinated forms of managed care.

PHOs

Unlike PPOs, which fail, almost by definition, to quality as organized systems, PHOs could do so, at least in principle. But most don't do so yet. Often organized by specialists or hospitals, they may lack a willingness to accept new paradigms and to direct more focus and funds to primary care. In most cases, physicians may remain only modestly committed to the system, and perhaps distrustful of hospital leadership. Additionally, unless linked to other PHOs, a one-hospital PHO will probably not provide the geographic breadth required to service employer group contracts.

The structure may not be inherently flawed, however, and—as was discussed in Chapter Five—older PHOs appear to be moving in the direction of increased integration. Specifically, they are merging with other PHOs to form super-PHOs and hospital systems, moving toward closed as opposed to open (any-willing-participant) physician panels, and directing more resources to primary care.

Many observers still believe, however, that hospital-based leadership will continue to limit the capacity of most PHOs to achieve the attributes of an ODS. Thus some recommend that hospitals encourage their staffs to form medical groups that may be affiliated with but independent of the hospital, and that those groups be given real leadership in the system. This is not a matter of physicians making better leaders; it is more a concern that hospitals will often fail to provide the most appropriate leadership for the purposes at hand.

Independent Practice Associations and Network Models

Until very recently, these HMO forms, especially the traditional IPA-type association of independent physicians, would have made few lists of organized or integrated systems. Many invoked aggressive capitation strategies and focused on primary care. But most were viewed as lacking capacity to coordinate care or to achieve high levels of communication between system parts. Few had system ties to hospitals, and—because participating physicians generally served a number of systems—physician integration and overall system focus were likely to remain at very modest levels.

Many of the new physician-organized HMOs assume this model. Clearly, such efforts take physician members beyond the organizational level of the PPO. But many, especially those organized by medical associations and financed disproportionately by specialists, are still likely to admit all willing providers. And most continue to pay by discounted fee-for-service, although a withhold of some form is generally invoked, as the network itself is at risk.

However, as outlined in Chapter One, some of these HMO forms seem to have achieved higher levels of coordination and physician integration in recent years. They have been invoking much more aggressive management styles, achieving dramatic reductions in utilization, and looking much more like membership medical groups than loose affiliations of independent providers. Some, in fact, have been organized by and remain linked to large medical groups with considerable capacity to manage physician practices.

Additionally, the IPA/network-type model can be strengthened by cementing ties between system organizers and a core group of primary care physicians via equity relationships, employment relationships, purchase of practices, or contracts that guarantee high patient volumes from the system. In this way an IPA/network model can increase emphasis on prevention and on coordination of care over the full continuum of services.

Finally, two unique advantages of the IPA/network approach—plus a one-time liability that may no longer be such a liability—should be noted. First, the models offer one of the easiest means of expanding (or reducing) numbers of physicians as needed to service an HMO's enrolled population and provide the broader geographic coverage where necessary. Second, at a time when more HMOs and ODSs are seeing advantages in contracts as opposed to employment and ownership relationships, the IPA/network approach has some particular value. Finally, given the ease with which information can be processed and moved today, limited communication and information movement capacity that once hampered the dispersed HMO models is no longer such a liability.

In the end (as noted in Chapter One), the IPA/network debate is in part a definitional one. The more modern IPA that features many of the attributes of the ODS is fundamentally different from the traditional loose affiliation of independent practitioners.

Some More Integrated Systems

Although clear-cut demarcations between less and more integrated delivery systems may not exist, some organizational forms clearly have greater capacity to achieve ODS goals.

Large Medical Group: Primary Care or Multispecialty

Increasing numbers of analysts view the large medical group as the core element of the ODS. It is clearly capable of assuming responsibility for care and risk (especially if it purchases reinsurance or is not directly responsible for all hospital risk). It can focus attention on primary care and foster higher levels of physician commitment to the overall system. These groups may also promote physician group-hospital integration via longer-term contracts with hospitals. For example, HealthCare Partners (a multispecialty group in Los Angeles) has contracts with a number of hospitals, but particularly with the downtown Los Angeles California Medical Center.

The multispecialty group may have the greatest potential to promote physician integration and coordination of care across a continuum of services providing, at least, that the numbers of specialists are appropriate, and that their organizational influence does not undermine a primary care focus. Integration may also be enhanced when the group has some central facilities that encourage group interaction. However, as information systems improve, this last factor may be of declining significance.

Still, while large medical groups may serve as cores of an organized system and may even lead it, they will generally require partnerships to fulfill some system needs. Except when very large, they tend to lack management expertise, including insurance expertise. Additionally, without longer-term contractual or other relationships with hospitals, they may lack capacity to promote integration in physician-hospital relationships or to bring a greater systemic focus to the hospital portion of the care continuum. Above all, they may lack capital for expanding facilities and for investment in information systems.

As discussed earlier, the partnerships required can and do come by way of relationships with hospitals, MCOs, or physician management companies. For example, the Sacramento Sierra Medical Group is affiliated with Sutter Health, which operates a number of HMOs. The Sharp Rees-Stealey Medical Group in San Diego is affiliated with the Sharp hospital system. And the Friendly Hills Medical Group was recently acquired by Caremark, a physician management company. With such partnerships in place, these group-centered systems can look much like some of the larger systems outlined later.

The Large Multispecialty Hospital Clinic

These entities can be distinguished from large medical groups by a number of factors, but most significantly in terms of system building by their affiliation with a major hospital. Thus many of the nation's best-known medical clinics—Mayo, Scripps, Cleveland, Sharp—are combinations of medical groups and hospitals (sometimes more than one hospital per group).

Some view these clinics as—potentially at least—the ultimate in organized systems. Their capacity to coordinate care, evoke physician commitment to the group (most physicians work on a salaried basis and only for the one group), and to foster a system focus can be extremely high. So, too, may be the capacity to promote collegiality, internal communications, and continuous quality improvement. For example, physician recruitment procedures in such organizations are generally very rigorous, aimed in large part at assuring both quality and proper fit with an organizational culture. Additionally, these institutions often function as academic health centers, enhancing their claim to high quality, especially on cutting-edge technologies and high-risk–high-cost cases.

But many of these institutions (including other major multispecialty clinics that offer HMOs) have had to make (or will need to make) significant adjustments to meet market demands in the new managed care environment. Most important, many are specialty or hospital driven, a circumstance sustained in large part by the organization's reputation for high-quality and high-tech care. Additionally, as is often the case with academic health centers, these institutions may be accustomed to fee-for-service payment mechanisms and to charging more than other providers; more than MCOs may be prepared to pay for some services.

Thus, high-tech, high-quality histories may produce complications as well as reputations. Given their leadership, and their focus on high-cost, high-tech care, adjustments to managed care paradigms emphasizing prevention and primary care can come slowly and painfully. Today, many of these clinics are making those adjustments—purchasing primary practices, expanding outpatient facilities, seeking longer-term managed care relationships, and so on.

Multispecialty Clinics and the HMO Connection

Some multispecialty clinics have taken a further step of providing their own HMOs. The Lovelace Clinic in New Mexico, the Fallon Clinic in Massachusetts, the Geisinger Clinic in Pennsylvania are all examples of such efforts. In these systems, medical group, hospital, and HMO are generally all part of one system. The Geisinger system thus includes an HMO with 125,000 enrollees, two hospitals, and a medical group with 500 physicians in forty-five sites. The Fallon system includes a clinic with 300 physicians, has 160,000 enrollees in its HMO, and owns a 483-bed hospital.

Like the multispecialty clinics described earlier, these organizations will serve patients in many health plans, in addition to those enrolled in their own system-sponsored plans. Thus, for example, 55 percent of revenues to the Fallon Clinic-owned hospitals come from non-Fallon system sources ("Friendly Hills Sold . . . ," 1994).

But as organized systems, such institutions may have a significant advantage over the multispecialty clinic that is not affiliated with an HMO—namely, a greater focus on the delivery of managed care services. The prominence of the HMO in the system may generate more organizational emphasis on prevention, primary care, and reduced utilization.

Multihospital Health Care Systems

Increasingly prominent in the ODS universe are large multihospital health care systems. These are not just HMOs, hospital systems, or multispecialty clinics, although they may include such. Rather, they are systems offering many products and services and accepting many forms of payment in many different circumstances.

But here an important distinction is required. Most hospital systems, as outlined earlier, are not ODSs. Few would consider Columbia/HCA hospitals, for example, to represent an ODS; the same would be true of a regional network of Catholic hospitals. Above all, such hospital systems generally lack a tie to a physician component. Without that component, consisting of more than a first-stage PHO, a hospital system or network cannot achieve maximum capacity to service managed care contracts.

Which is not to deny, of course, that such networks can achieve higher levels of coordination within their own systems and in performance of their hospital functions. Nor is it to ignore that one or more of their hospitals may be affiliated with ODSs in a given region. It is simply to emphasize that true coordination of care over a continuum of services requires a physician base, and perhaps even a semicommitted and integrated primary care physician base.

Many hospital systems, on the other hand, including the Utah-based Intermountain HealthCare System, the Henry Ford system in Michigan, the Sutter system in Sacramento, or Sharp Health-Care in San Diego (reportedly about to enter a joint arrangement with Columbia/HCA), achieve substantial levels of integration, and are often cited as models of organized systems. These and other multihospital health care systems have firm linkages with physicians—through staff or affiliated group relationships. They are increasingly focused on seeking managed care contracts, and many—like the Henry Ford, Sutter, and Intermountain systems, own their own HMOs.

Most of these systems have been in operation for some time. But others have evolved more recently, such as the Advocate Health System in Chicago, which formed out of a merger between the Lutheran and Evangelical health systems and which now includes seven hospitals, a medical group of several hundred physicians, and six PHOs ("Stephen M. Shortell . . . ," 1995).

Compared with the smaller systems described earlier, these systems are likely to offer more diversified services and products. These might include their own HMO product (perhaps a staff or group model), but also an IPA with physicians under contract, as well as PPOs and POS plans. Moreover, they will own not just several hospitals, often including at least one academic medical center, but medical facilities of several types. As of 1993, the Sutter Health system in Sacramento, for example, offered a variety of managed care plans, and included fourteen hospitals, six affiliated medical groups, skilled nursing homes and long-term care facilities, two surgical centers, and two community clinics.

In spite of their breadth of services and products, however, such systems may strive for and achieve significant levels of integration including physician and clinical integration. Medical groups affiliated with them often have exclusive relationships with the system. Sharp, Intermountain, and other such systems are often recognized as leaders in utilization management, and several of these systems have developed and implemented protocols and information systems throughout their systems, even where—as in the case particularly of Intermountain—the small rural hospital providing service may have few if any managed care contracts.

Because of their multiple products, facilities, and locations, such systems will employ different ownership and contractual relationships in delivering different services to different systems in different communities. And, perhaps because component parts of the system are so diverse in product and operational style, it may be difficult to achieve the level of system integration that a one-hospital multispecialty clinic or staff model HMO can achieve. Indeed, to address such concerns, some of these systems, like the Advocate System in Chicago or Intermountain in Utah, have begun to function and organize themselves as regional clusters of a larger system.

As might be expected, though, these systems are hardly without liabilities. Some, reportedly, suffer from excess hospital capacity, a lingering commitment to the hospital as a revenue center, and a reluctance or inability to downsize. Additionally, some analysts have suggested that such large systems have difficulty focusing on both hospital and medical group endeavors and would be better off focusing primarily on one and obtaining the other via contracts (Robinson, 1995). And while physician affiliates in such large multifunction systems may feel committed to the system unit to which they are attached, it may not be possible or even relevant for them to focus on outcomes of the system overall.

The Classic Group or Staff Model HMO

These models (Group Health Puget Sound, Kaiser, Health Insurance Plan of New York) remain the classic integrated systems, at least by most definitions. Of all the systems outlined, they are generally the most committed to managed care, in that most function in an almost exclusively managed care environment and treat patients mostly if not exclusively from their own system. Not surprisingly, they place the greatest focus on primary care and prevention, and their medical groups or staffs tend to reflect a more appropriate (for managed care) balance between primary care physicians and specialists than most delivery system organizations. The group and staff model HMOs also tend to stress development of an organizational culture, physician integration, exclusive relationships with providers, and more extensive use of protocols and clinical guidelines, all associated with higher levels of integration.

Interestingly, however, as discussed earlier, their growth in recent years has generally been modest at best. Although perhaps able to grow in terms of numbers of covered lives, many have only been able to maintain their share of the HMO market. In the view of many analysts, this may suggest that at least some organizational elements often associated with higher levels of integration come with a price tag of some kind. Specifically, the achievement of high levels of integration via exclusive contracts and employment of physicians may lead to reduced incentive and productivity. Additionally, the higher levels of integration that may attach to ownership of facilities (and a supposedly greater capacity to coordinate care over the continuum of services) may produce an excess of "bricks and mortar." Especially in times of widespread excess capacity of specialty services and hospitals, contractual relationships may have advantages over ownership. Finally, even the presence of an organizational culture may become a burden, especially in times that require change or downsizing.

How Much Integration?

The combination of a marketplace in rapid transition and a blossoming variety of organizational forms has led, among other things, to a healthy (spirited and positive) debate on both the merits of attaining various levels of integration and on the ability to attain them through contractual or networking relationships as opposed to ownership and employment relationships.

At times, to be sure, this debate can assume a straw man element. Most systems today are moving toward mixtures or hybrid forms that entail both ownership and contractual relationships. On one end of the continuum, Kaiser is invoking more contractual relationships; on the other end, as we have seen, IPAs and even PPOs maintain established ties to more organized groups and systems.

Nor is the debate about the value of the ODS itself. While analysts may debate the value of specific components of such a system the focus of current debate is not usually about the coming prominence of ODSs or even the goals associated with them. These are widely accepted. Rather, the debate is about the means by which those goals may be achieved. Thus the debate is not over whether coordination of care along a continuum of services should be improved, but over whether such improvement can be achieved by partners or contractual relationships rather than providers in the same system.

In large part this becomes a debate over the form that vertical integration or coordination should assume and over the value of different types of vertical relationships. Few challenge the reality of horizontal consolidation among physicians, hospitals, and health plans. While these trends certainly raise antitrust and other issues, most analysts see a certain economic inevitability, and even considerable value in at least some degree of horizontal consolidation.

As suggested earlier, the debate can be divided into varieties of questions or categories, three of which have been noted already: the nature of ties between the insurer and the delivery system, the degree of exclusivity between sets of providers and the delivery system, and the value of ownership versus contractual relationships or of one featuring economically integrated elements versus one based on contractual partnerships. A review of the cases for more or less integration focuses on these issues, as well as some others.

The Case for Higher Levels of Integration: A One-System Approach

Flowing from the logic of the organized system, the case for more integration emphasizes the goals of strengthening physician integration and clinical coordination across the continuum of care. Results from the most systematic study to date on integrated systems suggest that physician integration and clinical integration are interrelated. It is impossible, researchers concluded, "to achieve any measurable level of clinical integration for patients without a close relationship of physicians with an organized delivery system" (Shortell, Gillies, and Anderson, 1994, p. 53). Physician integration, in turn, was associated with such factors as the extent to which physicians identify with a system, use the system, and participate in its planning, management, and governance, all of which clearly go to the matter of exclusivity in the physician-system relationship.

Many analysts also associate improving physician and clinical integration with improved collegiality, greater use of in-house education efforts, more extensive use of protocols, and more rigorous physician selection and retention procedures. All of these attributes or processes tend to be associated with more highly integrated systems.

The logic of integration emphasizes the value of aligning incentives among providers, and assumes such alignment can mitigate conflicts among primary care physicians, specialists, and hospitals. Theoretically, at least, to the extent their focus is on the same bottom line, the system will be more likely to achieve the goal of utilizing the most appropriate and most cost-effective provider at all points along the continuum of care.

And there is some evidence that all these factors may contribute to higher performance levels of more integrated systems. Shortell and his team of researchers, for example, found that on a number of measures, including inpatient productivity, the integrated systems they are studying have better overall performance than less integrated competitors (Shortell, Gillies, and Anderson, 1994). Moreover, much research over the years has documented the success of the most highly integrated systems—group and staff model HMOs—at reducing utilization and overall costs. (More recent anecdotal reports, admittedly, suggest similar if not more impressive results in less integrated organizations.)

Most important, some advocates of higher levels of integration assert that such systems can achieve higher levels of quality. To date, however, that assumption may rest more on logic and expectation than on demonstrated proof. But at least from a consumer or marketing viewpoint, more integrated systems—including insurer-owned delivery systems—may have an advantage in capacity to demonstrate quality. Where insurer and delivery system are one—as, for example, in group or staff model HMOs or major multispecialty clinics with their own HMOs—consumers may be better able to evaluate quality of the delivery system, even if only by reputation.

By contrast, where the insurer has a contract with a provider network or system it doesn't own, including perhaps one that is, in turn, subcontracting with different sets of providers, both demonstrating and assessing quality can become a much more complex task. Even if the insurer can stipulate the specific delivery systems to which the consumer would have access, the consumer's information burden is still considerable. The same holds true for a marketplace in which most insurers are contracting with most provider groups. Assessing quality offered by insurers in such a marketplace may be not only difficult but meaningless. In such circumstances, assessing quality becomes a much more complicated, provider-specific endeavor.

Moreover, to date at least, more highly integrated delivery systems have demonstrated greater capacity to generate the kinds of data on which health plans might be compared (National Committee for Quality Assurance, 1995a). IPA-type arrangements and even many network or group-based models may be much less far along in developing such capacities. Even should systems and networks of all types improve such capacities, the quality of care in less integrated, more contract-oriented plans would still be harder to assess. Data in any given year might reflect performance of past contractors, not necessarily the current ones.

Still another argument for higher levels of integration focuses on the high costs of modern information systems. All agree that institution of such systems—which may entail expenditures of tens of millions over several years—will be mandatory in the new marketplace. But will those capable of undertaking such investments be prepared to do so in the absence of, at minimum, a very long-term arrangement? Will, for example, an insurer or hospital system install complex, expensive, and proprietary computer systems in the group offices of physicians who may, now or in the near future, contract with other systems or plans?

Finally, there is a public health aspect to the issue. In some respects, the gains in lower utilization and reduced health costs that systems of several types have achieved may be just a first stage, even the easier stage, in cost reduction. The next stage may focus on more embedded health risks in the population—such as drugs, alcoholism, smoking, sexually transmitted disease, crime, and poor nutrition. To some extent, the larger a system gets, the more willing it may be to invest in educational and preventive efforts to address these costs. If nothing else, the costs of such efforts will be spread over a larger base of premium dollars. Additionally, systems may be willing to undertake such investments—the benefits of which may accrue only over long periods of time—only when they are confident they will reap the benefits of them. Such benefits may only emerge when a system maintains a relatively stable patient population. Systems relying on contracts, and thus perhaps more likely to experience more sizable changes in patient population, may see fewer rewards in such public-health–oriented endeavors.

The Case for Contractual and More Flexible Systems

Few make a case for less integration. Most perceive value in integration. Those who may perceive more value in contractual relationships—in partnerships rather than systemic unity—believe that many, if not all of the goals of the integrationists can be achieved via more flexible relationships, including those that can be more easily terminated when they don't work out as planned.

This viewpoint rests largely on the value of flexibility and innovation in a fast-changing marketplace. In industries across the country, the talk is of right-sizing, outsourcing, and contracting. Bigger is not necessarily viewed as better, especially when it comes to vertical relationships that create complexity, more managerial challenges, and fewer obvious economies of scale.

In the health care industry, where excess capacity is the rule and reduction in utilization a primary goal, ownership of hospitals and long-term contracts with employees, it is asserted, may reduce flexibility and generate more liabilities than assets. If, for example, a contract-oriented health plan like US HealthCare were to lose enrollment, it could drop contracted providers or reduce the flow of patients to some providers. But should a staff model HMO like Kaiser lose enrollment, adjustment may require more difficult and painful choices. Laying off long-term employees or reducing salaries may be almost impossible, and the same number of beds are still in the same system-owned hospitals.

Moreover, the employment relationships inherent in many highly integrated systems may, it is argued, stifle individual productivity. So, too, may vertical relationships in a system, which, as noted earlier, may render it more difficult for individuals to associate with the organization's bottom line. And while organizational culture may be an asset, it may come with a price in insularity and reluctance to accept new paradigms.

Moreover, while more highly integrated systems, especially those entailing vertical relationships, may seek to increase coordination and to more completely align incentives to reduce conflicts across the continuum of care, a case can be made that some conflict and inherent tension are beneficial, whether between primary care and specialty physicians or between physicians and hospitals.

The less-can-be-better argument appears particularly compelling to many in light of the current system's excess capacity. With hospitals functioning at less than two-thirds of capacity on average, and managed care and risk-sharing strategies substantially reducing the numbers of specialists required in a network, contractual relationships have considerable appeal, especially to MCOs. This may be the case even if contractual relationships entail some decline in the ability to coordinate care, establish and enforce protocols, or promote physician commitment to a system.

But herein is the hub of the case: Most of those advocating more flexible contractual relationships do not believe such relationships need entail such losses, especially if the focus is on long-term partnering relationships rather than short-term, spot-market contracting.

Thus, an insurer like PacifiCare can have a long-term, even mutually dependent, relationship with a delivery system like Sharp HealthCare (Robinson, 1995). A medical group like HealthCare Partners may contract with a UniHealth hospital and maintain leverage over it (and thus some ability to align incentives) by virtue of its ability to contract elsewhere. The hospital, in turn, may still derive system benefits—but from its hospital system, not its physician-group partner. A major medical group may contract with physicians (rather than employ them) for service in a network or IPA, while still imparting to the relationship at least some of the benefits (protocols, communications systems, utilization management) of participation in an integrated system.

Thus long-term partnering may achieve virtual integration, without some of the reduced flexibility and other costs of actual integration.

Clearly, there is not likely to be a winner in this debate, not at least for some time. More likely, many flowers will bloom, involving experimentation with all kinds of possible arrangements and hybrid arrangements. Indeed, as we shall soon see, one of the possible contributions of public policy is to encourage such a flowering, or at least, to reject policy initiatives that might stifle it.

A review of the integration debate, however, does suggest an interesting potential relationship among integration, price, and quality. The case for increased levels of integration would appear to rest largely on matters relating to quality and quality improvement. By contrast, the case for more flexibility and contractual relationships appears to rest more on efficiency and financial performance. The current trends toward contractual relationships may imply, as was noted earlier, that price rather than quality has the upper hand in today's marketplace.

Leadership and Leverage in the ODS

Given the multiple types of systems likely to emerge, and the differing levels of integration they may pursue or achieve, what are the major assets and liabilities of MCOs, hospitals, and physicians in positioning themselves for leadership roles or exerting leverage in those systems? And what are the key choices they may face in pursuing those roles?

Assets and Liabilities of MCOs

As is the case with hospitals and physicians, MCOs—be they HMOs or traditional indemnity insurers now marketing HMO or other managed care products—have a series of clear assets and liabilities in the changing marketplace.

Most prominently, they have more control over covered lives. While such control ultimately rests with employers, MCOs are the primary general contractors in the insurance marketplace, especially when it comes to HMO products, which virtually all employers still purchase through insured arrangements. As a result of their general contractor status, these organizations also tend to possess overall management expertise in such areas as contracting, managing and bearing risk, marketing, and integrating large systems.

Additionally, as we have seen, MCOs are likely to have national as opposed to just regional structures, which can better enable them to achieve economies of scale and to promote national identification and reputation. And in the competition to reduce costs and utilization, these organizations may be advantaged, relative to physicians and hospitals, in greater willingness to make necessary delivery system downsizing decisions. After all, these tend, at least in their initial stages, to offer profit to the contractor and threat to the provider. Moreover, especially as compared to hospitals, MCOs (especially those that don't own hospitals) may be less inhibited in downsizing activities by community ties and complications arising from nonprofit status. Finally, but hardly least important, MCOs—especially those that are larger and operated for profit—have greater access to the capital required to expand via acquisition and to invest in management and information systems.

The liabilities of MCOs may lie mostly in history and perceptions of possible futures. While many now promote their role in coordinating and delivering care, the public traditionally views that function as residing with the physician. Many MCOs—especially traditional commercial insurers—are often viewed as distant from and lacking expertise in delivery of care. At best, consumers view them as organizations that pay the bills; at worst, as organizations that *don't* pay the bills, or that have an interest in restricting choice and access to care. Even the patient who understands the logic of managed care will generally prefer that the physician rather than the MCO be the coordinator of that care.

Looking ahead, some MCOs may suffer from a value-added problem. As ODSs form, and as they grow larger and more capable of managing care and capitation, there may be increased questioning—by those systems and by employers—of why 15 percent to 20 percent of premium dollars need flow to organizations not directly involved in delivering care. From the perspective of the ODS now assuming risk and managing care, the insurer should be passing on the 8 percent to 9 percent it once kept for performing tasks now being transferred to delivery systems.

Thus, the coming emergence of the ODS raises critical questions about the role of the MCO. Undoubtedly, many underestimate the complexities and costs of marketing, contracting, actuarial, managerial, and other services MCOs provide. Still, doubts will be expressed, and other organized competitors may see value in fueling those doubts, or in absorbing the insurer and general contractor roles.

As a result, many MCOs face a choice. They can assume for themselves direct responsibility for the organization and delivery of care. Alternatively, they can serve primarily as insurance and management companies—providing contractual, managerial, informational, actuarial, and marketing services to delivery systems that have responsibility for delivery and management of care. Clearly, such a decision can be made, and often is, on a market-by-market basis, with companies perhaps choosing the latter role where the organization is well established and the former where most covered lives are already spoken for.

Assets and Liabilities of Hospitals and Hospital Systems

Despite their obvious overcapacity problem and ongoing reductions in utilization, hospitals remain profitable. In 1993, hospitals averaged 4.4 percent profit, with profit levels increasing during the first half of 1994 to 5.9 percent. Significantly, in terms of leadership of organized systems, those hospitals in systems were particularly profitable, with operating profits rising 7.5 percent in 1993. Particularly noticeable was the 24 percent rise in operating profits in for-profit systems (Greene and Lutz, 1994).

Hospitals have kept profits up, even in times of declining utilization, by cutting expenses, tightening hiring practices, and improving management. Many have also undertaken substantial efforts to offset declining patient revenues with revenues from other ventures, such as outpatient surgeries and diagnostic imaging centers (Slomski, 1995).

Because they remain profitable, and because many maintain considerable financial reserves, many hospitals (especially for-profits) have the financial wherewithal to fund investments in organized systems, including the costs of securing a primary care base. For-profits clearly may be advantaged, both because they may have easier access to capital, and because they may be less encumbered than nonprofits by rules limiting the ability of nonprofits to shift tax-favored funds to physicians. Additionally, should they choose to do so, hospital systems have the capacity to form HMOs and compete directly with insurers; alternatively, if given regulatory permission, they could seek to contract directly with employers.

Many hospitals—especially major tertiary centers—have considerable managerial expertise, and a long lead over physicians in system leadership. Dozens of hospital systems already exist, and most are consolidating and raising levels of organizational integration. At least half of all hospitals now employ physicians or are affiliated with medical groups (Slomski, 1995). Moreover, many hospitals have launched prodigious efforts to strengthen physician relationships by purchasing practices and establishing PHOs.

In most communities, hospitals also retain political, public, and economic stature. Such standing may keep some open that should close; but it can also be an asset in terms of public credibility and status in marketing hospital-based systems, or in pursuing contracts with MCOs organizing such systems. Few MCOs (which may be well-known, but not greatly appreciated) or physician groups (with a handful of exceptions) have such an asset.

As potential leaders of organized systems, however, hospitals also bear obvious and significant liabilities. Above all, while they possess the finances and management skills to lead, such leadership may remain saddled with conflicts of interest. In the case of hospitals, at least, leadership and downsizing may not be the perfect fit. Nor may hospitals—even those embracing the new paradigm—be the most appropriate leaders of a system that will need to move dollars from hospitals to outpatient services, home health care services, and primary care.

These conflicts may be even more apparent as stress on hospital revenues continues and perhaps worsens. If hospital utilization continues to fall toward the numbers achieved by the most efficient systems, and if (as seems likely) Congress enacts significant reductions in Medicare payment rates, revenue pressures on hospitals will intensify. Theoretically, such pressures should move them toward greater acceptance of new paradigms; but perhaps less so, or more slowly, when those new paradigms threaten their long-standing practices, or even their existence.

Declining utilization will also compound the hospital excess capacity dilemma. With many hospitals functioning at 50 percent capacity or less, both MCOs and physician groups may see more value in short-term hospital contracting than in longer-term partnering relationships with hospitals.

Hospitals are also facing stiff competition from physician-led networks and large physician groups. Physician management companies are also emerging as formidable competitors, offering physicians managerial skills, capital, and perhaps security, while leaving them substantial autonomy in physician practice. As detailed in Chapter Five, hospitals have made major efforts to secure ties to primary care physicians, but many observers remain skeptical of the integrating capacity of the PHO.

Assets and Liabilities of Physicians and Physician Groups

As noted earlier, in the context of the ODS, primary care physicians possess very substantial opportunities and assets, but they may experience difficulty in deploying them. This may be a case, then, of being in the driver's seat of a Mercedes, but without the resources to fuel the tank, and with competitors already around the first turn. Especially where they are inexperienced in managed care relationships, physicians may enter the competition in a defensive mode, limiting their ability to organize until too late. Many specialists, of course, face particularly stark scenarios, and more limited opportunities in the ODS.

The great asset of primary care physicians and groups is the growing consensus that they are the most appropriate hubs for emerging delivery systems. They are best positioned to manage and oversee care across the continuum, and they are best positioned to promote prevention. Most important, especially when judged against specialists or hospitals, they are (or at least should be) less threatened by the demands of managed care and organized systems (including lower utilization of higher-cost services and providers, and more emphasis on greater use of the most appropriate, cost-effective provider).

Which is not to ignore the argument of some that greatly increased emphasis on primary care may go too far. Indeed, some analysts believe the managed care burdens being placed on primary care physicians are excessive, especially given their lack of training for such management. Some also believe that specialists could be more appropriately utilized—often for more frequent consultations with primary care providers—or for primary management of chronic illness.

The opportunities for primary care physicians are most apparent in the stiff competition among hospitals, MCOs, and physician management companies for their services and commitments. The current undersupply of primary care physicians in many maturing markets only enhances such opportunities, although such undersupply is likely to disappear, at least in most metropolitan markets, in the relatively near future. Indeed, in some markets primary care physicians are already finding themselves part of an oversupply.

The need to lock in primary care physicians, when combined with the perception of their role as hubs in the new systems, has led many to focus on the need to place physicians in leadership roles in those systems. Thus, many more progressive hospitals are seeking to maximize physician board membership in PHOs. And legal entities like foundations, management service organizations, and joint ventures involving physicians, MCOs, and hospitals are structured to provide physicians leadership roles or numbers of board members above what their financial contribution to the venture may justify.

But physicians may not always be trained or prepared to assume or take advantage of leadership opportunities. They are not members of large institutions and thus suffer from far greater levels of economic insecurity. Their medical school training did not focus on the business and marketing decisions with which they

are now confronted. And the nature of their past business relationships have left them in conflict-oriented relationships with
many of those with whom they may now need or want to partner—
most notably hospitals and insurers.

As for most state and county medical societies, as well as the
AMA, these have rarely been at the forefront of the managed care
movement. They tend to be dominated by specialists, and by older
physicians less accepting of new realities. Many of the organizational efforts launched by those organizations have been defensive
(for example, support of open-panel physician networks) or anti
managed care (for example, support of any-willing-provider laws).

Most important, physicians tend to lack capital and—with the
exception of some larger groups—management expertise. Even
sizable groups, as has been noted, have had to turn to larger corporate partners for expansion or installation of new information
systems. Their lack of management expertise may be multilevel,
applying both to the management of the individual practice or
group (witness the dramatic growth of physician management
companies) and to the management of larger, integrated systems.

The lack of management expertise should, of course, decline
with time. But overall, most analysts expect that primary care
physicians will need larger corporate partners. Those are clearly
available. The difficulty for physicians is to decide which partner
to choose, what goals should be held paramount, and under what
circumstances.

Specialists, of course, face more unpleasant pressures. The level
of oversupply in most specialty services is great, and not likely to
decline significantly in the near future. And with traditional laws
of economics asserting themselves, it is already becoming apparent that oversupply does not enhance market power or leverage.
Even membership in multispecialty clinics may not provide an
answer. Many of these are attempting to reduce their imbalance of
specialty to primary care providers—and the larger physician
groups emerging outside California are reportedly more primary
care centered than some of their California prototypes.

As a first response to the new environment, many specialists
have sought expanded access to managed care revenues through
the establishment of IPAs, medical-society–originated HMOs, and
PHOs. Unfortunately, however, the catch-22 of these efforts is that

their chances of prospering are inversely related to the degree of influence specialists assert in them.

Specialists are also turning to the establishment of carve-out specialty networks. And given today's emphasis on contracting, some of these may prosper. Organizers of managed care plans, as was discussed earlier, appear increasingly receptive to capitated contracts with such specialty groups and networks—whether formed to deliver just one service, such as cardiology, or a full continuum of specialty services.

Specialists may also find it valuable (as encouraged in some managed care environments) to consider changing roles and relationships with primary care providers—serving in more educational and advisory capacities that increase contacts between physicians but decrease referrals of patients who may not truly need specialty care.

But, almost inevitably, larger and more painful adjustments may be in the offing for many specialists. Unlike hospitals, where reduced revenues can be at least temporarily offset with decreased costs, many specialists are likely to experience a more direct connection between lower revenues and lower incomes.

The ODS and Public Policy

The evolution of the ODS will depend far more on its reception in private markets then on decisions of public policy makers. Still, the rise of the construct raises some issues that those policy makers may be required to address. It may also raise some opportunities for cooperation between government and private interests.

Among other things, policy makers may wish to (or be forced to) review actions that may have the impact of easing or inhibiting the development of organized systems. As noted in our analysis of horizontal and vertical integration efforts, so-called anti-managed-care laws may be relevant here; so, too, may be laws or regulations pertaining to direct contracting between employers and organized systems, and to scope of practice, which may excessively limit the capacities of organized systems to use the most appropriate and cost-effective providers. These are discussed primarily in Chapter Nine.

Issues of quality also seem especially relevant here. Governments (as well as private employers) wishing to promote quality and competition on quality may need to address data collection and other matters that would facilitate the capacity of employers and consumers to choose plans based on quality—and thus encourage those plans to promote and improve quality. Policy makers may also need to address the extent to which government involvement and leadership are necessary in promoting quality improvement efforts such as outcomes research, or development of clinical guidelines that may be either beyond the capacity of private plans functioning on their own or not of significant enough market value for plans to undertake on their own. These issues are discussed in Chapter Eight.

Policy makers must also review ways in which public responsibilities and public facilities may be affected by the emergence of more organized systems. It may be asked, for example, if the new private systems will incorporate public systems, and if they do not, what will be the impact on the public systems and those they serve? Such questions may raise concerns for public responsibilities, but also opportunities. For example, as organized systems grow larger and more comprehensive, and especially as many seek to enroll Medicaid recipients, the goals they need to serve—prevention, improving population health status, even reductions in health-care-associated costs of violence, drug usage, and sexually transmitted disease—may begin to overlap with the goals and definitions of public health. Opportunities for cooperation in these areas could be well worth exploring. These issues are discussed in Chapter Ten.

Part Three

Private Markets and Public Interests

Chapter Seven

After the Clinton Plan
Relying on the Marketplace

Whatever it might have turned out to be, the Clinton administration's health care policy team didn't set out to create a "big government" health care plan. In fact, the core assumption underlying the plan was that while government intervention might be required to make health care markets work, the marketplace, rather than government intervention, would represent the true driving force of reform. Lower prices and higher quality would come via increased competition—driven by stronger, smarter purchasers—between private health care organizations. In this sense, administration policy accurately foresaw the coming of market change and intended to encourage rather than constrain it.

A number of policy decisions, however, combined to obscure core administration goals and strategies. As the Clinton plan moved from concept to legislation, the elements of government intervention, regulation, and restructuring—and certainly the appearance thereof—seemed to expand in proportion and significance, opening the door to the "big government" attack that proved so devastating.

The Road to Big Government

To some extent, the reality and appearance of government restructuring and intervention might have been avoided or mitigated by different policy or political choices. But in part it may have been unavoidable, dictated by basic reform needs, political realities, or legislative rules.

167

First, to level the competitive playing field and thus foster competition on price and quality, as opposed to risk selection, the legislation had to include a series of insurance reform rules. These reforms were, it should be emphasized, also part of most Republican proposals. But they did impose a series of new rules and levels of government intervention.

Second, the administration—in its original reform formulation, at least—pushed the purchasing cooperative concept more aggressively than necessary, mandating that large numbers of consumers access the insurance marketplace through such cooperatives. Administration policy makers never envisioned the cooperatives as having the power, over any one or any thing, that opponents ascribed to them. And, in fact, although they had considerable responsibility, it was responsibility to enforce rules imposed by others. In short, they had very limited power of their own. But they were a new institution, and the selling of new institutions takes time, especially when associated with government. The administration, in a tactical error, probably compounded the problem by misnaming the cooperative a *health alliance*. The term had no descriptive value, and the plan sorely needed clarity. The terminology also created an image of conflict when security was to be the main theme of the reform effort.

But far more important than the name was the failure to acknowledge how controversial the cooperatives would prove to be, and how many of the same purposes might have been achieved (albeit less effectively and less efficiently) without cooperatives, or at least without mandating them. The concept, without question, was the right one; but so much so that it probably needed only a good push and not a set of requirements.

Third, the administration's goal of universal coverage led to a seemingly unending set of rules and legislative demands: rules for coverage of the uninsured; rules on who would have to pay how much and to whom; rules to make certain that, now that government was mandating the purchase of insurance, burdens of that purchase would be spread equitably; rules on subsidies to those who couldn't afford to pay; rules that would minimize the extent to which low-cost states would subsidize high-cost states; and many others. Which, again, is not to suggest that the universal coverage goal was wrong. It wasn't. But achieving the goal did require a host of government-established rules—more, perhaps, than policy makers had anticipated—that played into the big government argument.

In the end, a guarantee of quality care for all (insurance coverage for most, something else for others), rather than universal coverage, would have been easier to achieve. It would also, of course, have been far less compelling, and less of a guarantee to the uninsured and those who might become uninsured, in other words, virtually everyone else. Additionally, a more modest goal may have been unacceptable to many of reform's most ardent and loyal supporters, to whom universal coverage had become the sine qua non of health care reform.

Fourth, given deficit concerns and budget rules, the administration could not create an open-ended entitlement. The belief— held by many administration policy makers—that market forces might render specific spending caps less necessary, was irrelevant. Congressional budget rules, deficit projection requirements, and a variety of political forces mandated a guarantee that costs would not rise above projections. That guarantee would require an additional and controversial set of statutory requirements (opposed vigorously by insurers, providers, and many others) relating to restraints in the growth of health care spending. The administration's core theme of health security—again, the right theme— compounded the problem. If the program didn't offer a financial guarantee that it would work—that is, if it didn't impose some regulatory limitations on spending—what kind of security could it offer? Thus the choice: more security and more regulation, or less security and less regulation.

Fifth, and finally, the administration's plan was exceptionally broad, ranging far beyond universal coverage or even restraints in cost. Policy makers, in a sense, tried to rationalize the system. They correctly understood relationships between parts of the system and when one part had to be adjusted to achieve primary reform goals, they tended to adjust the other part as well. Thus, the scope of the reform plan inevitably and continually expanded, somewhat like a reapportionment map in which changes in one district mandate changes in others. Clearly, doing less, even if it meant leaving some inefficiencies in place or some problems for future policy makers to resolve, would have been the wiser choice.

Health Care Policy Today

All that being acknowledged, however, the big government label, while perhaps offered up on a platter, was also a mislabel. Those who employed it to defeat reform probably used it more than they believed it. In the end, it wasn't really big government that they or others feared. It was any one or many of the myriad changes reform might legitimately produce, or at least that opponents claimed reform might produce. Opposition groups developed around such things as higher costs to businesses or insured individuals, declining profits to some insurers, public spending to assist those unable to afford health insurance, loss of choice of physician (clearly a misplaced fear, as the Clinton plan guaranteed more such choice than most of us have today), reductions in health care spending that might affect individual or organization income or profit, and so on.

There were, of course, many other reasons for the failure of the reform effort. The issue of "big" or too much government was only one. But whatever the causes of failure, it now appears highly unlikely that major national interventions to guarantee care for all will be undertaken in the near future.

But some things don't change. Health care spending still amounts to a seventh of the national economy. For most people, concerns about their ability to pay for and gain access to high-quality care remain, as they always will. The federal and state governments still have massive health care responsibilities—including Medicare, Medicaid, and other public health programs. Finally, although less obvious to many, the nature of the insurance business compels government attention. Those insured need long-term guarantees that insurers will be able to deliver as promised, and the nature of the business is such that more profit is generally made when less is paid out, creating an inherent tension between insured and insurer. As a result, insurance has always been, and will always be, a heavily regulated industry.

Added to these constants is the reality of dramatic change, as we have attempted to describe it, in today's health care marketplace.

It should come as no surprise, then, that while health care reform has died, health care policy remains on the government front burner—as it always will. Indeed, many of the issues remain the same as when the Clinton administration undertook its reform effort. There is just one exception: no one is talking very much about coverage for the still-growing numbers of the uninsured.

Maintaining a Competitive Marketplace

With the rejection of national health care reform—and with it, most likely, the rejection of increases in government regulation of health care markets—the nation is, intentionally or not, putting its health care eggs into the basket labeled marketplace competition.

By most accounts, to mix metaphors, the basket has a good chance of bearing fruit. Intense competition ignited in part by expectations of reform are continuing well after the end of the reform effort. The health care marketplace is changing rapidly and most would suggest that the changes occurring—while sometimes disruptive and unsettling for many—are overdue, and offer potential for both lower costs and higher quality.

At the core of that marketplace change is the reality of consolidation. As outlined in several of the preceding chapters, it is occurring at all levels and among all actors, including physicians, hospitals, and insurers, and, at least as important, among buyers as well. Without question, most of this consolidation, like other changes, is long overdue. The health care marketplace has long been marked by fragmentation of both sellers and buyers, poor coordination, and many other cottage-industry-like trappings.

For the most part, such consolidation does not—according to both policy analysts and antitrust enforcers—threaten competition. As one economist noted, all CEOs "may desire monopoly power, [but] the miracle of modern capitalism is that none are able to keep it and hold it for more than a moment" (Robinson, 1995).

In fact, most analysts today believe that consolidation in the health care sector is likely to enhance competition, or at least to promote higher levels of efficiency among competitors. In some limited numbers of circumstances, however, consolidation can endanger competition—threatening higher prices or lower quality. When it does, market forces need the backup of government intervention, generally in the form of antitrust enforcement.

In any case, because so many eggs are in the marketplace competition basket, and perhaps specifically because consolidation activity is so intense, a core goal of government policy must be to make certain that market forces work. The big may need to get bigger—but not too big. Finding the right level of tolerance for consolidation may or may not mean government intervention. But, unquestionably, it puts the economic spotlight on antitrust policy and its implementation in the health care marketplace.

In this chapter, we shall review the critical significance of antitrust policy in that marketplace. We shall also look at some other means by which government policy might encourage or at least protect a healthy competitive environment. We begin with a review of the consolidation issue: just how concerned should we be about the consolidation now so evident in the marketplace? Under what circumstances might that consolidation prove to be procompetitive or anticompetitive?

One Perspective: Oligopoly Fears May be Inflated

If substantial consolidation in today's health care marketplace has been and is inevitable, generally procompetitive, and yet also at some point a threat to competition, the obvious question becomes: How much consolidation is too much? When does horizontal or vertical consolidation among providers and MCOs produce such high levels of market power that competition is undermined?

Analysts offer different answers to these questions, and those answers can lead to advocacy of different policy positions. But there appears more consensus around these questions than might be expected. All recognize the potential for oligopoly and for anticompetitive collaboration in at least some markets. But most economists and other knowledgeable observers continue to believe, that, at least in large markets, most merger and consolidation activity is still procompetitive—or at least not anticompetitive—and that various market and other forces are likely to keep the potential for anticompetitive consolidation in check.

Such analysts will certainly allow that aggressive antitrust enforcement may be required in some circumstances, and that the threat of that enforcement is a powerful inhibiting factor on anticompetitive action. But most—including antitrust enforcers—clearly envision antitrust as the backup, believing that enforcement powers should be invoked very selectively and cautiously, and that considerable amounts of consolidation can go forward before the antitrust button need be pushed.

Many even hold this view with regard to markets as consolidated as Minneapolis, where consolidation trends—including dramatic reductions in numbers of MCOs and delivery systems—have been most pronounced (Office of Technology Assessment, 1994; Kralewski, 1995).

A number of assumptions appear to underlie this view: for one thing, analysts note that there may be no greater economies of scale in health care delivery than there are in most other economic sectors. The shift from a fragmented to a consolidated health care industry may be occurring at an unusually rapid pace. But the speed of that consolidation reflects the prior state of fragmentation—and perhaps the past effectiveness of some physician organizations in maintaining it—not some extraordinary set of circumstances that will lead to uniquely high levels of consolidation in health care relative to other industries.

Indeed, trends in the nonhealth industries suggest, if anything, that firms can grow too large. At some point size may inhibit innovation, generate complications rather than improvements in coordination of individuals or units, render motivation of employees more difficult, or produce a variety of other unproductive processes or outcomes (Robinson, 1995).

A full exploration of pros and cons of firm size is beyond our scope here. But there is enough downsizing, outsourcing, contracting, and other such arrangements occurring in health care and other industries to suggest that growth in firm size is not inevitable, and may in fact have its limits.

Of course, a distinction must be drawn between economies of scale and market share. A hospital system, for example, may conclude that there are no more economies of scale or profits to be achieved by adding a seventh hospital. However, they can still be expected to maximize market share for the six hospitals, and depending on the market such efforts and positioning might still lead to dangerous levels of market share and power for the system. Moreover, firms or systems of even very modest size can pose threats to competition in smaller communities. The point here, then, is hardly that firms or systems will magically stop growing when their market share or power reach dangerous proportions. It is that there is no inevitability to the expansion of firm size.

Exclusivity and New Entry

Tendencies toward anticompetitive behavior or configurations may also be restrained, some assert, by the predominance, in most markets at least, of nonexclusive contracts between MCOs on the one hand and provider systems and networks on the other hand. In such markets, provider systems, rather than having exclusive contracts with one MCO, are likely to contract with several. Indeed, as discussed earlier, provider systems such as large multispecialty clinics may even operate their own HMOs while also contracting to have their providers service competing systems. Figure 7.1 compares the two types of relationships between plans and providers. Such nonexclusive contractual arrangements, the argument suggests especially when combined with the existence of excess capacity in provider systems, create system capacity that can be put to work elsewhere, preserving competitive options, including the critical option of new entry for both MCOs and providers (Nichols and others, 1995).

When the prominence of POS options (which as will be recalled are growing rapidly) are added to this mix, fluidity in the market is further enhanced. Patients have greater capacity to move between providers, who, in the absence of exclusive contracts with another plan, are available and prepared to serve them.

Nonexclusive relationships may predominate even in markets like Minneapolis and San Diego, where consolidation of both MCOs and providers has been substantial. In Minnesota, which now has just three major insurer organizations, there has even been a significant amount of vertical integration between MCOs and delivery systems. HealthPartners, for example, merged with Ramsey HealthCare, and the Medica HMO (itself a consolidation of HMOs) merged with HealthSpan, a hospital system, to form a new system called Allina.

Still, in Minneapolis, as in San Diego, most MCOs contract with many if not most provider systems. Such circumstances may result, in part, from the prominence of major community delivery systems and the belief of MCOs that their marketing will suffer if they do

Figure 7.1. Exclusive/Nonexclusive Insurer/ Provider Relationships.

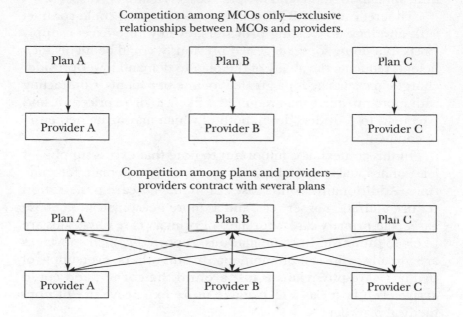

Competition among MCOs only—exclusive relationships between MCOs and providers.

Competition among plans and providers— providers contract with several plans

not offer access to all those systems. Thus, in San Diego, MCOs may feel compelled to contract with Scripts, Sharp, and the University system. Exclusive contracting may also be inhibited by the demand of employers and individuals for substantial choice of physicians and provider systems. Such a demand will require an MCO to contract with a large number of physicians and provider systems; exclusive relationships with such large numbers is not economically viable.

Among other things, the absence of exclusive ties between MCOs and providers—especially when combined with the prevalence of excess capacity—tends to ease burdens of entry for new MCOs, a critical element in keeping markets competitive. When more providers are both available (excess capacity) and free to work (in nonexclusive contractual relationships) there is more free capacity with which to combat anticompetitive action. Indeed, it was concerns about preserving options for new entry that, in part at least, prompted Minnesota to enact legislation barring such exclusive relationships between plans and providers, except in the case of group or staff model HMOs. Three health plans with exclusive provider relationships, it was feared, could inhibit competition, stifle innovation, and increase costs (Hellinger, 1995).

Theoretically, an MCO seeking market control could contract with and lock up existing providers, even where excess supply exists. But doing so, as suggested previously, could be highly inefficient, reducing the ability of the plan to demand lower provider charges in exchange for a greater volume of patients. Contracting with more providers than required is likely to drive prices up, and payments to providers down, both of which may invite new entry of competitors.

In this context, it is important to note that excess supply—at least of hospital beds and specialists—is likely to remain for some time. Additionally, as increases in managed care penetration reduce utilization of services, and as more new physicians choose careers in primary care, shortages of primary care physicians are likely to diminish. In some markets, reportedly, such shortages are already historical phenomena. In still others, oversupply of primary care physicians is just around the corner, and could arrive even faster as MCOs make more expansive use of non-medical providers.

Finally, those with less concern about the widespread likelihood of consolidation leading to anticompetitive behavior note the capacity of purchasers to maintain and generate competition. Large employers, including public employers and employer coalitions, have a considerable capacity to engender competition among MCOs, among providers, and even between the two.

Purchasing cooperatives, for example, can increase competition between insurers by offering new market entrants or other insurers low-cost and direct access to consumers. Competition between provider groups can also be encouraged—as is now envisioned in Minnesota—by instituting direct contracting between employer coalitions and delivery systems with individual consumers choosing a delivery system rather than an insurer. Finally, competition between plans and delivery systems could be encouraged by allowing both to compete for enrollees, as envisioned in some 1995 Medicare reform proposals. Such competition (as well as direct contracting arrangements), might require an adjustment of regulatory requirements defining circumstances under which delivery systems should be defined as or allowed to function as insurers.[1]

A Second Perspective: Concerns about Oligopoly

Even those who generally view current market trends toward consolidation very positively recognize the real potential of various kinds of consolidation activity to yield anticompetitive outcomes. If nothing else, all recognize that the development of some degree of oligopoly is inevitable in some communities. The issue, in these cases, is not whether it will happen, but what to do about it.

Above all, it is clear that some of the forces—nonexclusive contractual relationships, excess capacity, even prominence of POS plans—might diminish or change with time.

As was discussed in Chapter One, one reason for the continuing prominence of less integrated (and unusually nonexclusive) IPA-type managed care forms is that excess capacity offers advantages to those employing shorter-term contracting with shifting groups of providers rather than longer-term and often less flexible contractual arrangements.

However, as excess capacity diminishes, and as managed care penetration and consolidation increase, exclusive contracting may have greater relative appeal. Indeed, in its first "snapshot" report, one Robert Wood Johnson project suggested that exclusive contracting was more common in high-penetration markets (*Conference Participants*, 1995). The rise of the ODS could also increase the prominence of exclusivity in relationships between providers and delivery systems, as these systems are more likely to embrace such relationships. Thus, the combination of consolidation in and organization of delivery systems, increases in managed care penetration, and declines in excess capacity could yield increases in exclusive contracts and declines in free capacity. Such developments, taken together, could yield a very different competitive environment from the one envisioned in the more fluid scenario outlined earlier.

Those particularly concerned about threats to competition also focus on the newly emerging hospital systems. Many such systems

---

[1]This issue will be discussed both later in this chapter and in Chapter Nine.

and joint ventures, it is suggested, may be structured to expand cooperative activities while staying below antitrust enforcement thresholds. If nothing else, these systems are spawning a wide variety of degrees and types of collaborative activity—horizontal (among hospitals) and vertical (between hospitals and physicians)—which may put great strains on antitrust enforcement resources and analytical tools. (See discussion of antitrust, later in this chapter.)

Additionally, some express concern regarding the potential leverage of some physician groups. If trends toward larger group practices accelerate, and if more physicians establish exclusive relationships with physician groups, some of these groups—especially in small and midsized communities—may emerge with sizable market shares and dangerously high levels of market leverage. (Such arrangements, of course, could come under the purview of antitrust enforcers.) Dominance in a community of a few exclusive physician networks would render new entry by MCOs more difficult. New entry by independent physicians may also prove to be more limited in the near future. As one Federal Trade Commission representative recently noted, decreasing numbers of physicians coming out of residency programs appear able and willing to start new practices (Steptoe, 1995).

A related concern noted by several observers, comes in the form of de facto exclusive contracts between physicians and MCOs. Under such an arrangement, a physician or group of physicians would not actually sign an exclusive contract with an MCO, but would in fact serve only that organization. Such de facto contracts could represent (illegal) efforts to avoid detection by antitrust enforcers, which would be more likely if the exclusive nature of the contracts was apparent. If successful, the result of such efforts would be less opportunity of new entrants to win physician contracts and enhanced market leverage for existing MCOs or provider networks.

Still another concern about loss of competitive environments stems from the current perceived rush to dominate markets undergoing rapid transition. Such markets are reportedly distinguished by particularly aggressive competition among highly capitalized MCOs to secure access to and control over primary care providers, many of whom are insecure and ill prepared for the pace of change. In such circumstances, purchasing of practices and other contractual arrangements can result in markets that get locked up, and quickly, with new entry very difficult. Again, such activity could be subject to antitrust scrutiny; but the pace and scope of market change can produce uncertainty as to whether or not a threat to competition exists. This, as will be discussed later, may be especially true given strained enforcement resources and limited experience of enforcers in analyzing impacts of certain kinds of market changes and conditions.

Activities of some states to immunize specified activity from federal antitrust enforcement is also of concern to some. Under federal law, states may take such action only if there is a clearly stated policy to replace competition with regulation, and if the state actively (not just by statute or potential) supervises the activity in question. For example, Maryland state law exempts hospital mergers, joint ownership of medical equipment, and other activities providing they are approved by the state's Health Resources Planning Commission (Polzer, 1995).

In recent years, there has been what one researcher labeled a flood of antitrust exception legislation in the states (Polzer, 1995). Between 1992 (when the U.S. Supreme Court issued a major ruling on the subject) and early 1995, twenty-two states passed laws seeking to immunize a variety of collaborative arrangements between health care providers. And according to at least one authority, both private parties and public entities are becoming more aggressive in seeking to use state immunity laws to insulate themselves from antitrust enforcement in a wide variety of merger, networking, or negotiating activities (Bloch, 1995).

Undoubtedly, the growth of immunization activity in states reflects the dramatic growth in consolidation-related activity in the health care sector. It also may reflect the relative strength of provider groups at the state level. Since most provider groups are state rather than federally regulated, their political resources are generally more targeted into state legislative efforts. State legislators may, as a result, be more receptive to provider appeals.

Whatever its causes, the rise of state antitrust immunity legislation is of concern to some. For one thing, the passage of many such laws could lead to excessive variation in antitrust statutes across states, and therefore to overall antitrust enforcement problems. Additionally, there is a fear that some immunity legislation will be either inappropriate or, as a result of provider pressures and weak regulatory structures, enforced with less than ideal levels of aggressiveness. Concerns are expressed, for example, that states may grant antitrust immunity for specified provider activities (for example, hospital partnership activities) without providing adequate regulatory means to control or reduce potentially anticompetitive effects of those activities (Bloch, 1995).

Others, it should be emphasized, take an alternative view of state immunity laws. They note that many have been only recently approved, that there is limited experience with them, and that there is considerable uncertainty as to the acceptance of many such laws in federal courts. It is also argued that most antitrust attorneys will advise clients that if their activities are not, in fact, anticompetitive, it is generally easier to comply with federal rules than to subject themselves to new sets of state regulations and supervision.

But whichever view is more accurate, state immunity laws can complicate the antitrust picture. In doing so they reinforce the concern of many that the pace, scope, and complexity of change may complicate the task of protecting the marketplace from anticompetitive activity.

These concerns result, in part, from the sheer scope of activity, and the ability of antitrust enforcers to monitor it. But they also reflect concerns about the ability of enforcers—in the absence of systematic research on a host of new relationships—to assess the impacts of the various components of market change, and thus to determine the need or lack thereof for antitrust intervention.

To this general concern, some add a more clearly policy or even political concern; that the potential impact of market change is so great that public responses to that change need to reflect broader policy direction than that which can come from enforcement agencies and antitrust policy.

Antitrust Policy and the Health Care Marketplace

It is probably fair to say, without any negative aspersions intended, that the first step in the consideration of joint venture, merger, or other consolidation activity, is the hiring of an antitrust attorney. MCOs, hospitals, physicians, pharmaceutical companies, and others have all had to question whether or not their activities might entail antitrust violations.

Some such activities might be "per se" violations, considered to be so clearly anticompetitive that it is not necessary to determine if anyone was harmed by the action, as with price fixing, market allocation agreements, or boycotts. Alternatively, collaborative efforts can be evaluated and rejected or restrained under the "rule of reason" analysis. Under such an analysis, antitrust enforcers weigh the potential threat to competition and prices (via enhanced market power) of a new collaborative arrangement against the potential benefits of that collaboration—for example, lower cost or improved efficiency—for consumers.

Antitrust Enforcement

A review of recent antitrust agency enforcement actions, speeches, and guidelines, and of the views of knowledgeable observers of those activities, suggests several conclusions. First, the agencies—specifically the Federal Trade Commission (FTC) and the Department of Justice (DOJ)—have been very hesitant in taking action to restrain or block consolidation activity, generally viewing most such activity as procompetitive, or at least not on balance anticompetitive.

Second, when it comes to consolidation activity, the focus of enforcement has been, and should be, on providers as opposed to MCOs. Most observers, like the agencies, tend to view most consolidation activity among insurers as imposing no serious threat to competition.

Third, the agencies have gone to considerable, probably unprecedented, lengths to assist system actors in trying to predict how potential collaborative arrangements might be evaluated and judged.

Fourth, the most controversial area of antitrust enforcement policy relates to the activities of nonintegrated, non-risk-sharing physicians attempting to form networks and negotiate prices.

Finally, most knowledgeable observers appear to agree with the priorities and policies of the enforcement agencies; but some express concern about the scope of responsibilities involved and the capacity of enforcers to accurately assess potential impacts of various developments and thus effectively oversee a highly volatile marketplace.

Consolidation as Procompetitive

Overall, antitrust enforcers have reflected the analyses offered by most economists that the great majority of consolidation activity in the health care sector does not, at least on balance, threaten competition—and may, in fact, offer consumers benefits in increased competition, lower costs, greater efficiency, or higher quality. While those considering merger or acquisition activity often complain about antitrust complications and limitations, intervention by antitrust enforcers has been relatively rare. Indeed, the Physician Payment Review Commission (PPRC) concluded that "enforcement records of the agencies indicate that they have been less aggressive in challenging health care related activities than is generally perceived" (Physician Payment Review Commission, 1995, p. 295).

* *MCOs:* The agencies have generally refrained from interfering with plan mergers, even those involving large organizations and market share.

* *Hospital joint ventures:* Neither the DOJ nor the FTC have challenged a hospital joint venture (Bloch, 1995).

* *Hospital mergers:* Between 1981 and 1993 there were 397 hospital mergers, just 68 of which resulted in a preliminary investigation—and only 15 of which were challenged (Physician Payment Review Commission, 1995). To be sure, in response to the recent increase in merger activity, the number of agency investigations has increased in recent years. Between spring 1994 and spring 1995, the FTC initiated enforcement actions to block four mergers of acute care hospitals. But, as an agency representative emphasized, the increase in investigations does not reflect a change in policy, or in the view of enforcers that most mergers do not threaten competition (Steptoe, 1995).

* *Physician networks:* There have been very few challenges to the formation of physician-sponsored networks. In fact, as of 1994, the agencies had never challenged a legitimate physician joint venture[2] (Physician Payment Review Commission, 1995), such as a

---

[2]A legitimate joint venture is determined by the existence of certain attributes. One key issue is whether or not the endeavor involves shared risk. Even if a joint venture is considered legitimate, it may still be evaluated under the "rule of reason" approach to determine if anticompetitive impact may outweigh procompetitive aspects.

PPO, PHO, or joint purchasing arrangement. Some organizations of physicians, however, most notably the AMA, continue to vigorously assert their view that the antitrust playing field is uneven, and that it restrains the emergence of physician networks that would be procompetitive.

Unique Focus on and Advice for Health Care Sector

Given the unique level of merger, acquisition, and other collaborative arrangements occurring in the industry, enforcement agencies have made a considerable effort to offer guidance to potential collaborators.

In 1993 and 1994, the enforcement agencies produced health care policy statements addressing issues in hospital mergers, physician joint ventures, provider information exchanges, multiprovider networks, and nonexclusive physician networks. The agencies also promised to issue advisory opinions in ninety days. Additionally, they outlined safety zones, within which collaborative actions would generally be viewed as acceptable, and outside of which they would be subject to a case-by-case analysis. Thus the safety zones do not define the limits of acceptable behavior. Indeed, collaborations that did not fall within the zones have gone unchallenged (Whitener, 1995).

It is widely acknowledged that the breadth and detail of this advice is beyond that afforded actors in any other economic sector.

Antitrust and Physicians

Currently, perhaps the most controversial (although not necessarily the most important) area of antitrust policy has been that focused on the formation of physician networks. This policy area has been controversial for many years, with the agencies consistently objecting to efforts by physicians, whom they view as horizontal competitors, to engage in price fixing, boycotts, or efforts to undermine alternatives to traditional fee-for-service medicine (Whitener, 1995).

Many physicians and their associations remain critical of these enforcement practices. Most recently, they have argued before state and federal legislatures, as well as the agencies, for greater physician

flexibility to combine efforts of unintegrated physicians in negotiating fees with MCOs. The antitrust playing field, physicians assert,
is not a level one, with physician-organized networks and insurer-
organized networks being treated differently, resulting in a chilling
effect on the ability of physicians to organize networks that might
be beneficial to consumers.

Specifically, physicians object that when networks they form do
not undertake either substantial integration, including the sharing
of risk, or certain technical steps to have third parties negotiate fees,
their efforts to negotiate prices are viewed as collaboration among
competitors (that is, as price fixing), and are likely to be judged a
per se violation of antitrust law. They argue that if the same network
of physicians—also not sharing risk—is organized by an insurer, the
insurer is allowed to establish fees without being charged with a per
se violation for doing so. Rather than be viewed as per se violations,
physicians assert, their networks should be judged according to the
rule of reason, or on whether or not the network is actually anticompetitive. Where such a network is not anticompetitive, physicians assert, it should be allowed to go forward.

Physicians make a similar argument with regard to current
guidelines on the percentages of physicians who can participate in
a nonexclusive network—that is, a network that contracts with a
number of plans. Specifically, they object to the suggestion that
networks run antitrust risks should they involve more than 30 percent of physicians in a community, and 20 percent if the network
is exclusive. Physicians acknowledge here that the mere listing of
a safety zone percentage doesn't mean the network is in violation
of antitrust law. They assert, however, that such a listing has a chilling effect on network formation.

Finally, physicians assert, they need more ability to organize to
resist efforts of MCOs with increasing amounts of market power to
drive down physician rates, even to the point where quality could
be jeopardized.

Viewed from some perspectives, the physicians' case has some
merit. In its 1995 annual report, the PPRC expressed some sympa-
thy with physician concerns, suggesting that antitrust market share
rules could be discouraging the development of physician-led organizations and networks. And if, in the age of consolidation and
minimal government regulation, public policy needs to encourage

competition and the formation of varieties of competing systems, then a case can be made for letting a thousand flowers bloom, including those that may be planted by physicians. This may be especially true in the case of physician-led networks. As discussed earlier, many analysts of organized systems believe that physician leadership of such organizations is to be encouraged, and that even unintegrated networks can be a step in the right direction.

On the other hand, there is a difference between encouraging the formation of genuine physician networks, which integrate, share risk, and promote efficiency and innovation, and encouraging physician networks the main purpose of which may be increased market power and the main effect of which may be higher prices. Current antitrust rules appear to allow for considerable amounts of physician collaboration, even in the absence of integration. These include joint purchasing arrangements, data exchanges, and network formation that invokes a third party negotiator (called the *messenger model*). Few such arrangements have been challenged.

Far more substantial collaborative efforts, moreover, can be undertaken when accompanied by integrated arrangements. As outlined earlier, many such networks are forming today—as group practices, even as HMOs. Admittedly, some are having trouble organizing or competing. But the primary causes of their difficulties are not antitrust rules; they involve capital, management expertise, and a variety of other factors.

Thus it remains far from clear that providing physicians greater antitrust leeway to negotiate as non-risk-sharing networks will do much to facilitate true physician integration or the formation of physician-led health care delivery systems. Indeed, in the view of some, granting loose physician networks exemptions from antitrust rules might undermine physician incentives to form the stronger and more integrated types of delivery systems that may offer real consumer benefit.

As to the level-playing-field issue, a critical distinction must be made between the nature of horizontal (physician-organized) and vertical (insurer-organized) networks. The former is a relationship between competitors, the latter is between a purchaser and independent physician suppliers, in which there is some measure of public protection from the need of the insurer to get as low a physician price as possible. Physician-set network rates, it is feared, will raise the floors from which many negotiations begin, resulting in higher prices for consumers.

Additionally, it should be emphasized that if insurers were to join together in a horizontal relationship to cooperate in price negotiations, they would face the same antitrust scrutiny as that faced by physician collaborators.

As for the 30 percent rule, the antitrust agencies have made it clear in word and action that it is not intended as a limit on the size of a physician network—only as a floor below which networks are unlikely to be challenged.

Overall, then, while it may be wise public policy to encourage physicians to assume leadership in health care organization and delivery, it remains far from certain that antitrust rules create a chilling effect on such organization or leadership, or that antitrust exemptions will achieve those goals. Indeed, granting such exemptions might have the effect of encouraging anticompetitive behavior. As the PPRC concluded in rejecting the case for major revisions in antitrust policy, "The available evidence . . . is not sufficient to warrant creating safe harbors or other exemptions . . . for physician-sponsored networks at this time" (Physician Payment Review Commission, 1995, p. 284).

However, what cannot be won from the executive branch can sometimes be won from the legislative branch, and as of late 1995 it appeared possible that Congress might yet respond to physician appeals for antitrust relief. Additionally, Congress seemed prepared to allow physician networks to form—at least for providing services in the Medicare program—under different rules than currently apply to insurers or HMOs.

Antitrust and Hospitals

Like physicians, some hospitals and hospital associations have appealed for greater freedom from antitrust restraints. Specifically, some have advocated that they be allowed greater freedom to promote efficiency by dividing the performance of services, reducing duplication of facilities, and engaging in other joint activities and arrangements.

Additionally, some argue, hospitals should be allowed to consolidate negotiating power so as to strengthen bargaining positions vis a vis larger and more powerful payers, lest they be weakened financially. Excessive stress on financial viability, it is suggested, might cause a decline in quality or in the introduction of new technologies. It might also result in the closure of weaker hospitals, many of which might be those most likely to care for the uninsured.

But here, too, as in the case of physician concerns over antitrust enforcement, such views win only very modest support outside the hospital community. Supporters of current antitrust enforcement policies are quick to note, for example, that the DOJ and FTC have never opposed a hospital joint venture such as the provision of specialized clinical or expensive hospital services. The agencies have consistently concluded that on balance the vast majority of hospital consolidation activity is not anticompetitive (Steptoe, 1995). Moreover, enforcers have noted, the absence of risk-sharing does not necessarily suggest that such ventures will be viewed as anticompetitive.

In the case of mergers and acquisitions specifically, enforcers make very clear that the vast majority of these are not likely to be challenged. Such intervention will be limited to those few cases in which—even where there may be integration and risk sharing—trade-offs between greater efficiency and greater market share may still be negative for consumers. Thus, according to the DOJ, "The [Antitrust] division will challenge mergers where the merged hospital entity will have the ability to raise prices to consumers and the hospitals cannot demonstrate that efficiencies from the merger will outweigh any anticompetitive effects" (Polzer, 1995). Given such reasoning, the FTC, while not challenging the merger of Columbia and HCA, demanded that Columbia divest itself of Aiken Regional Medical Center in Aiken, South Carolina, because the new entity's market share there might threaten competition (Polzer, 1995).

As for the argument of some that relaxing antitrust rules on hospital collaboration will reduce duplication of facilities, most antitrust experts believe that a competitive marketplace is more likely to achieve such objectives, especially when those facilities do not offer competitive value. Thus, market forces will adequately perform the task of reducing duplication and inefficiency and, as a result, there is little need for government to relax antitrust rules—opening the door to anticompetitive arrangements—to achieve such goals.

Recently, it appears, hospitals have been less aggressive in seeking changes in antitrust rules. The American Hospital Association, reportedly, is largely satisfied with the new DOJ/FTC-issued guidelines (Serafini, 1994). The changed hospital attitude, some believe, may also reflect a fear on the part of the hospital community that hospital victories in antitrust policy would spill over into similar victories for physicians. Such dual victories might, it is suggested, result in a net loss to hospital bargaining positions.

Hospital Partnerships: Pushing the Antitrust Envelope

As noted earlier, however, the rise of hospital systems and partnerships is raising new and complex issues in antitrust policy. Activities of such partnerships can include such significant activities as purchasing, budgeting, coordination of clinical services, strategic planning, sharing of operating income and expenses, and perhaps most important of all, contracting.

Advocates of such efforts are likely to assert the goals of improved efficiency, lower costs, and other proconsumer objectives. But more skeptical observers are likely to apply the infamous "duck test," suggesting that the real purpose of much of today's partnering activity is to achieve the values of mergers or acquisitions without entering them, to reduce the probability that various activities will produce antitrust scrutiny, and to improve market power.

Whichever viewpoint is accepted, it seems clear that current market trends in the hospital sector may be generating more gray areas in which assessing the pro- or anticompetitive nature of a relationship can become more difficult. Evolving hospital partnerships—which increasingly include vertical relationships with physicians—evoke complex questions about relevant geographic and product markets, the generation of efficiencies, effects on competition and new entry in both hospital and physician sectors, and other factors relevant to the evaluation of marketplace change.

Antitrust enforcers make no effort to deny the significance of these new questions—especially those relating to emerging questions focused on systems and vertical relationships. They emphasize that they will review the actions, not just the specific legal structures, of the new partnerships. Above all, they suggest, they will attempt to ascertain whether partners are functioning as merged entities when it comes to negotiating with payers (Burda, 1995a). And most important, as noted earlier, they are quick to note their receptivity to new research and to guidance on appropriate approaches to such issues.

But such admissions, while accepted in good faith, do not necessarily assuage concerns of some with the state of antitrust capacity today, including the fundamental question of whether—in today's volatile marketplace—anyone can adequately project the impact of various developments on marketplace competition.

If nothing else, the pace of consolidation activity and the existence of so many gray areas may suggest a problem of resources. When increasing numbers of delivery systems, providers, and plans operate in antitrust gray zones, resources of antitrust agencies may grow strained. While the need for antitrust oversight has obviously expanded dramatically, agency resources have not. Thus some fear that even if antitrust policies may be appropriately constituted, the resources required to enforce them may be lacking.

With such concerns in mind, some question whether or not antitrust enforcers possess the analytical tools required for the task at hand, especially with regard to distinguishing between pro- and anticompetitive collaboration in the hospital sector. One study concluded, for example, that the new enforcement guidelines have proven to be only slightly helpful to enforcement agencies in deciding what hospital mergers to challenge—that is, they have limited predictive value (Zwanziger, 1995a).

Most specifically, questions are being raised as to whether or not antitrust analysis may have to focus more on systems than on individual actors, more on linkages between collaborators that do not involve ownership, and more on the complex web of relationships between types of market activity and their impacts in different market circumstances. (See, for example, Zwanziger, 1995a; Fubini, 1995.) In this context, it is relevant to note that antitrust enforcers and the guidelines they have established are noticeably more directed to horizontal rather than vertical integration, where enforcement agencies acknowledge they have "insufficient experience" (Polzer, 1995, quoting antitrust guideline statements).

Taking an even broader though not necessarily more critical view, some have begun to question the wisdom of vesting so much reliance in antitrust enforcement when many of the questions at hand are those of public policy, which ought to be addressed in legislative and political as well as legal and enforcement settings. It is one thing, it has been argued, to leave to enforcement agencies and the courts the role of evaluating trade-offs between efficiency and market power. But when trade-offs entail issues of quality, access to care, and costs of care for large populations, as well as specific impacts on such issues as the capacity of systems or communities to deliver charity care or the ability of academic medical centers to perform teaching and other functions, or the financial health of disproportionate share hospitals, debate over those trade-offs may deserve and require elevation to more visible and more public forums (Shactman and Altman, 1995).

The Potential for Oligopoly and Anticompetitive Behavior

It may follow from the foregoing analysis that attention and research on market competition issues—by both antitrust enforcement agencies and public policy makers—needs to focus on at least some of the following circumstances:

- When managed care and the networks it produces extend into smaller urban and rural communities.
- When and where excess in provider capacity is reduced or nonexistent or where exclusive contracting between MCOs and providers and within delivery systems is growing in prominence.
- In fast-maturing markets where MCOs may be engaged in efforts to secure primary care and other provider partnerships.
- At the provider—as opposed to the insurer—level.
- At the hospital partnership or strategic alliance level, where impacts of relationships, and even the relationships themselves may be unclear, and of near-infinite variety.
- At the potential impacts—on such factors as costs, efficiency, competition, and quality—of various vertical relationships.
- In the absence of strong purchaser coalitions with the capacity to encourage new entry of MCOs, foster direct

contracting with delivery systems, discourage excessive
consolidation of plans, or promote individual consumer
choice as a means to strengthen the position of providers
relative to plans.
- Where providers, especially, might deploy political strength to
gain immunity from antitrust enforcement that is not balanced by appropriate government regulatory action.
- Where POS options or indemnity plans, which give consumers
more options are less pervasive. Prominence of such arrangements may help keep some providers independent of networks, or may encourage networks to be nonexclusive, so
that providers in them can service more consumers.

Maintaining a Competitive Environment: Other Policy Options

From a policy point of view, in addition to highlighting areas of
concern that may justify more policy input or research, the list in
the previous section and the discussion preceding it suggest a few
particular actions public policy makers might consider.

They might, for one thing, assess the capacity of antitrust agencies to effectively monitor the high levels of partnership, networking, joint venture, system formation, and merger and acquisition
activity in today's marketplace. If resources are found to be limited,
additional investments here would seem fully appropriate.

Encouragement of purchasing cooperatives for both public
and private employees may offer policy makers another tool in
keeping markets competitive. These will be discussed in greater
detail in Chapter Eight. But among their other values may be a
capacity to employ their control of large numbers of insureds to
influence provider arrangements. Among other things, as noted
earlier, purchasing cooperatives can increase access of MCOs and
providers to insureds and to contracts. In this way, they may be of
assistance in keeping barriers to entry low.

Most organizers of purchasing arrangements, of course, may
not view this as a key employer or purchasing cooperative function.
Thus, employer coalitions may need some prodding and education here. Where relevant, government-run cooperatives could provide demonstrations of means for securing these goals.

Networks and Contracts: Some Policy Considerations

Policy makers also need to consider how various networking rules or contractual arrangements might affect marketplace competition.

For example, the list of antitrust focal points might suggest that support be offered to anti-exclusivity legislation. Minnesota, as noted, has passed such a law, and New Hampshire is considering one.

Both the Minneapolis case, an urban one, and the New Hampshire example, a rural one, may suggest that where competing MCOs are few, where excess capacity is small or nonexistent, and where exclusive contracts appear to threaten competition, some limits on those relationships may appear justified.

But support for such restrictions, absent compelling evidence of an anticompetitive effect, would seem highly premature, and generally violative of the goal of encouraging competition. Overall, there seems little justification for restricting the right of MCOs and providers to form exclusive relationships should they choose to do so. Indeed, many believe such systems will achieve higher levels of integration, improved quality, and lower costs.

The any-willing-provider concept, in which networks may be compelled to accept any provider willing to accept network rules, would seem even more clearly violative of competition enhancement goals. These laws will be discussed in more detail in Chapter Nine. But it is relevant to note here that such laws could restrict both the types of networks that may evolve in a market as well as the differences, in physician membership, between networks. As such, they can limit innovation and competition.

The same logic would appear to apply to other so-called anti-managed-care laws, such as those that limit the differences between co-payment rates faced by enrollees for network and nonnetwork providers or freedom-of-choice laws that guarantee individuals the right to reimbursable services from any qualified provider, even one not under contract to the managed care plan in which the individual is enrolled.

Clearly, some of these proposals offer apparent value as consumer protection. But, as in the case of the any-willing-provider laws, they may also harbor the potential to restrict innovation and competition. Except in the face of clear consumer protection needs, wiser policy might dictate that MCOs generally be free to adopt their own approaches to these issues. Such approaches may include, obviously, the increasingly common POS plan, which offers consumers greater access (at higher cost) to out-of-network providers. Indeed, the spread of the POS option suggests that MCOs are likely to adapt to meet consumer demands, and that the need for legislation limiting the freedom of plans to structure network options may be less compelling than once appeared to be the case.

Direct Contracting

Finally, policy makers may wish to consider—indeed, they may be compelled to consider—the values and dangers in direct contracting between employers, especially self-insured employers, and delivery systems.

This option is emerging from the growth of ODSs capable and desirous of accepting full- or partial-risk managed care contracts. Unquestionably, the option raises complex regulatory issues of if, when, and how to regulate or monitor delivery systems that may be assuming risk and taking on other insurance-type functions, without having to obtain licensure as an insurer. Additionally, the option raises controversial ERISA-related issues.

These regulatory and legal questions will be analyzed in Chapter Nine. But the direct contracting option also highlights issues of market competition and purchasing that range well beyond regulatory structures. For one thing, the option of ODSs, however defined legally, to market directly to employers might spur efforts to form such systems. Even more important, perhaps, the direct contracting option suggests the possibility that the focus of competition could be shifted from insurers to delivery systems.

It should hardly be surprising, then, that provider groups especially are stepping up efforts to win legislative approval of direct contracting options, and that MCOs are opposing those efforts with equal conviction.

Potentially, at least, direct competition between delivery systems, as opposed to MCOs, could offer significant advantages to purchasers. When choosing between insurers, purchasers may be forced to evaluate plans and networks, the quality of which may change as networks change, and the reputation of which may be difficult to evaluate. By contrast, direct contracting may offer options to contract with well-known, specific, and local sets of providers. For example, employers or consumers contracting directly with a Mayo Clinic or Columbia University Hospital system may be able to assess, by reputation if nothing else, the quality of care they will be receiving. Contracting, by contrast, with most MCOs (especially those that organize rather than directly deliver care), physician-organized networks, or IPAs may offer much less clarity. In this respect, a consumer is more likely to have relevant knowledge regarding a prominent regional hospital or large multispecialty group than of a network or IPA organized by a national managed care company or even the local medical society.

Competition on quality between such regionally identifiable delivery systems might be further enhanced if the choice of delivery systems was given to individuals—who may prove to be more quality conscious—rather than employers, most of whom remain primarily focused on price. Indeed, a case can be made that the arrangement most likely to encourage competition on quality is one in which individual consumers choose between delivery systems organized by locally known provider organizations.

Additionally, some argue, direct contracting will offer greater incentives to delivery systems to improve quality or lower cost. Where delivery systems are not capitated by insurers, the profits attaching to these improvements (for example, improved outcomes on complex heart surgery or protocols leading to earlier detection of breast cancer) may go, at least in the short term, to the MCO. Under direct contracting arrangements, by contrast, delivery systems would reap virtually all the benefit of lowering cost or raising quality.

The choice, of course, need not be competition between MCOs and insurers or competition between delivery systems. Theoretically, both could compete, with MCOs, where they chose to, contracting for delivery system components, and ODSs contracting for insurance services, including solvency guarantees. In this way, the kinds of arrangements between insurers and providers might grow more varied, potentially increasing levels of innovation and competition, as well as choice for employers and consumers.

Some advocates of direct contracting also envision substantial savings resulting from the presumed elimination of the insurance function and the administrative costs associated with it. Such anticipation, however, often erroneously assumes that integrated delivery systems, functioning alone, will somehow dramatically reduce costs in marketing, enrolling individuals, adjudicating claims, and guaranteeing solvency.

Moreover, it must be noted that many systems and employers seeking direct contracting opportunities assume that such contracting will enable them to function outside state insurance rules. These rules, viewed as limitations by many, include such provisions as mandated benefits, premium taxes, guarantee issue and renewal requirements, limits on the imposition of preexisting conditions, and, most important, limitations on the rating of groups according to their experience. To delivery systems and to some employers—especially those with younger and healthier populations—the advantages of contracting outside of such a regulatory framework may appear substantial. Whether it is in the larger public interest to allow or encourage contracting outside of those rules is a very different matter, and one that we will turn to shortly.

Chapter Eight

The Search for Value

When purchasers seek value, most consider both quality and price. Indeed, one common definition of value is quality divided by price. Thus, value rises as quality rises and as price declines.

Such a construct, of course, oversimplifies the issues at hand. For one thing, quality is often difficult to assess, especially when the purchase involves a package of goods—in this case benefits—as in the case of a health care plan. As for price, varying benefits—including deductibles and co-payments—can render comparisons more complicated than would otherwise seem to be the case, at least for anyone other than an actuary.

Still, the equation reminds us that value involves both price and quality and also that there is a relationship between the two.

From the point of view of today's health care purchasers, it is safe to say that price is the long suit. There is, to be sure, an unprecedented focus on quality and on the means of measuring it. But it is also true that purchasers (employers especially) appear more concerned with price, and that MCOs and providers have been more effective and more aggressive at reducing price than in improving and demonstrating improvements in quality.

In this chapter, we review how current market trends and the new partnerships may affect the potential of delivery systems to produce lower prices and higher quality, and means by which purchasers—with government assistance where necessary—may enhance that potential. As we shall see, the potential to increase value is clearly present and rising. Delivery system reform offers substantial promise in this regard. Rising also, it would seem, is the sophistication of purchasers and the strength of the demand side. But, as we shall also see, sophisticated purchasing of health care services and insurance is still in the maturing phase, and the ability to compare plans on value remains modest at best. Additionally, it is also clear that while the capacity to and interest in reducing price is actual, the capacity to and interest in improving quality remains much more in the realm of potential.

On Premiums and Purchasing

An assessment of the short-term future of costs and premiums has already been undertaken (see Chapter One), and need not be repeated in detail here.

Suffice to say, for our purposes here, that a reasonably strong case can be made that current marketplace changes are producing and will continue to produce a positive impact on health care costs and premiums.

Supply Side Changes

On the supply side of the equation, several elements appear to be most central. First is the rising penetration of prepaid managed care plans, many of which have demonstrated or are at least beginning to demonstrate a capacity to reduce utilization and costs. Second is the resultant rise of competition among those plans (as opposed to between those plans and fee-for-service systems). Research is revealing that rates of increase in costs of health care services in competitive markets have been slower than in less competitive markets. For example, as shown in Table 8.1, rates of increase in health care costs have been lower in California than in the nation as a whole. Moreover, the fact that rates of increase in California have been lower across all the services suggests that costs are not being shifted from one to the other. Third is the reorganization of the health care delivery system—including both consolidation and integration—which, offers the potential at least to generate greater productivity and value—providing, of course, that consolidation does not jeopardize the vitality of competition. While such reorganization is clearly a part of the overall movement toward more productive MCOs, it is also distinguishable from it.

The essence of these changes is not just the rise of competition; it the rise of competition between organized systems capable

Table 8.1. Competition and Health System Expenditures: Cumulative Growth in Real Per Capita Outlay, 1980–1991.

	Total Expenditure (percent growth)	Hospital Services (percent growth)	Physician Services (percent growth)	Drugs (percent growth)
United States	63	54	82	65
California	39	27	58	41

Note: Lower California rates of increase in all categories suggest that costs are not being shifted from one category to another.

Source: Zwanziger, 1995b. Used with permission of the author.

of improving performance. In a fee-for-service or even a PPO framework, when individuals can choose any provider and insurers possess only rudimentary means of controlling costs, competition is minimal in large part because there isn't much over which to compete. Insurers or purchasers can press for lower rates, improve efficiency in plan administration, add deductibles, expand or contract networks, and even implement more aggressive utilization review processes. But capacity (let alone drive) to improve competitive position by actually improving performance in the delivery of care is limited. (Which may explain, in large part, why the sometimes prodigious self-insurance efforts undertaken by some large employers usually bore so little fruit. They simply didn't have enough pieces to rearrange.)

By contrast, a competition between prepaid, organized health care systems is highlighted both by greater capacity on the part of competitors (as organizations) to improve and by greater need of—and reward for—doing so. In addition, in contrast with most fee-for-service or PPO networks, the modern prepaid health care organization offers purchasers something they can evaluate. There was never much to compare in a series of indemnity or PPO plans in which enrollees generally had the same options. But organizations differ and therefore provide more opportunities for comparison, which, for obvious reasons, enhances competition. In prepaid health care markets, this may be especially true because the price (premium) offered is fixed and because the benefits offered are fairly well standardized.

With the rise of competition, the capacity of health care markets to flout the traditional laws of economics has diminished. The excess supply, which once drove services and prices up, is gradually transformed into an asset of the demand side. As competition between MCOs for employer contracts increases, and as providers increasingly view themselves as dependent on managed care contracts controlled by those MCOs, leverage over providers increases, and excess supply begins to produce what theory says it should produce—lower prices. MCOs, prepaid delivery systems, and employers find they have the clout to pay less per procedure or hospital day, even as they reduce the number of procedures or days they pay for. In this way, it is important to note, MCOs become less like suppliers and more like purchasers. In many respects, they become allies of employers, shifting more influence to the demand side, and putting more pressure on the supply side.

Demand Side Changes

Looking back, these developments may have been inevitable. Yearly double-digit increases in premiums, based on traditional fee-for-service health care delivered by independent and largely uncoordinated providers, simply were not sustainable.

But this is not to suggest that purchasers—employers especially—played the role of passive observer. Many of the changes outlined above occurred (or at least occurred in more condensed time frames) in large part because of increasingly assertive efforts on the part of purchasers—most notably large employers—including, it should be emphasized, governments.

Much of the increased sophistication among purchasers and increased aggressiveness in purchaser efforts stemmed, no doubt, from the right of large employers to self-insure under ERISA. Between 1980 and 1985 alone, the percentage of self-insured group health business rose from 30 to 55 percent (Etheredge, 1995a). Undoubtedly, one of the values self-insurance offered was freedom from state insurance laws, including mandated benefits, premium taxes, and state regulation. Additionally, self-insurance offered large employers the opportunity to receive the full benefit of whatever expenditure reductions they could achieve, an opportunity that in turn inspired concerted efforts to increase their sophistication as purchasers and their clout (often in coalition) in the marketplace.

Whether they focused primarily on contracting with already established health care plans or networks or whether they went further to develop more unique arrangements, business managers of these self-insured employers began to demand that providers and organizers of plans do more than provide some volume discount; they began to demand greater efficiency. Drawing on a growing literature documenting wide disparities in utilization rates among both communities and provider groupings, they questioned utilization rates and began to request—and then to demand—justification for higher costs. The result was an increasingly sophisticated and knowledgeable large-employer purchasing force.

But, even as it grew more sophisticated, the self-insurance movement generated only marginal success. Indeed, health care costs were still soaring at the end of the 1980s, and, according to many reports, some of the largest self-insuring employers were acknowledging their limits—if not their failure—when it came to controlling those costs.

At almost the same time, however, it was becoming more apparent that, at least in some markets, HMOs were reducing costs and premiums. In the early 1990s, differentials between indemnity and HMO premiums began to increase. Surveys of employer costs began to show yearly reductions in the rates of increase in HMO premiums. Reports of employer coalitions (primarily government purchasers) in California and Minnesota winning reductions in HMO premiums made national headlines.

Even, then, as they saw value in self-insurance and in paying their own health care costs in (albeit better managed) indemnity and PPO plans, many large employers saw increasing value in prepaid health care. In effect, perhaps, they saw that others were doing it better. Today, many large employers appear to be concluding that it might be wiser to function as aggressive purchasers of plans run by others rather than as managers of plans they develop, contract for, and run on their own.

Such logic, of course, might direct the new breed of sophisticated large-employer purchasers (as it has in many cases) to a new compromise—stay self-insured for the benefits of that status while contracting with HMOs to deliver health care services. However, because prepayment to an HMO entails the transfer of risk to the HMO, HMOs are insured rather than self-insured products. As a result, purchase of an HMO product—according to insurance commissioners—subjects the arrangement to state insurance rules. To date, therefore, while considerable efforts are being undertaken to find the gray areas of the matter, self-insurance generally remains limited to payments for PPO or fee-for-service arrangements. In these arrangements employers can maintain risk and remain self-insured. But PPOs and fee-for-service are hardly the wave of the future in the new marketplace. As of 1993, of the over eighty million individuals insured by large employers (those with a hundred employees or more), two-thirds remained in PPO or fee-for-service plans, most of them self-funded (Hodapp and Samols, 1994).

The Rise and Value of the Purchasing Coalition

Emerging out of the recent experiences of large employers are two critically important purchasing tools: the purchasing coalition or cooperative, and the development of means by which MCOs and providers can be pressed to higher performance and evaluated on performance measures. These related trends and tools appear particularly relevant in the purchasing and evaluating of health plans purchased as insured products by employers. But they have also been important tools (especially where the pressure is exerted directly on regional providers as opposed to MCOs selling insured plans) for self-insured employers.

Today these coalitions may represent the benchmarks of employer purchasing. Not only can they pool demand-side power; but because of the rise of the organized system, they may be able to make better use of that power. It is not just a matter of pools driving market change, or of market change producing a response of pooling—it is also a matter of market change expanding the opportunities for effective pooling.

Specifically, the rise of managed care and organized systems offers purchasers and the pools they may create greater potential to demand, collect, and distribute more performance-oriented data from providers and plans (such information rarely exists in non-managed-care systems); to compare plans offering similar or identical HMO benefits on price; to select and compare plans to be offered by the coalition based on that data; and to require participating plans or providers to achieve various performance goals. In short, the purchasing coalition is well positioned to benefit from the rise of managed care and of the ODS environment and from the increasing competition among plans and providers that marks the new health care marketplace.

In their efforts to accomplish these goals (both successes and failures), the progress and approaches of these coalitions provide a critical window through which to examine current capacities of purchasers to increase value in health care purchases. The general potential of these coalitions is discussed in this section. The rising demand for performance-oriented data (and the rise of the accreditation movement) is noted here, but discussed in greater detail later in this chapter.

Employer purchasing coalitions—of which there may be as many as 150 today—assume many different forms, and pursue a variety of purchasing goals and strategies—including negotiating premiums, demanding and collecting data on plan or delivery system performance, purchasing plans for participating members, and issuing consumer satisfaction reports.

The largest group of coalitions represent mostly large self-insured employers. Some of these may contract with a number of managed care plans, offering the employers or employees of member groups a choice among those plans. Alternatively, coalitions may serve self-insuring employers by pooling employees and by contracting directly with providers from whom the self-insured employer then purchases services.

Two other prominent coalition types are those established by governments (numbering twelve at the end of 1995) to pool and service small employers, and those established by governments (most states and the federal government operate in this way) to pool their own employees. Technically, some of the latter are not pools; they may represent only one employer. However, their numbers and strategies are such that they function as large pooling purchasers.

The types of employer purchasing coalitions, the general strategies they employ, and the innovative approaches they have undertaken vary in many ways. The text boxes distributed across the rest of this chapter illustrate some particularly successful examples of coalitions at work.

Value and Tools of the Purchasing Coalition

Whatever employers they may represent, forms they may assume, or strategies they may pursue, most purchasing coalitions would appear to have several goals in common. These include the following: lower administrative costs, the opportunity to offer more choice of plans, an enhanced capacity to foster competition among MCOs on price and quality, and greater market leverage for participating members.

At minimum, coalitions can lower administrative costs, improve economies of scale and expertise in purchasing, and increase the market leverage of employer members. The larger coalitions are likely to have at least several full-time employees with increasing expertise in health care purchasing. And depending on size and role of the coalition, administrative costs can run as low as under 1 percent.

Small employers, obviously, who suffer particularly from high administrative costs in insurance transactions, may see particular value in these opportunities. But even most large employers, it should be emphasized, do not have enough employees in most markets to generate market power. And while there are obvious and well-known exceptions—Xerox, General Electric, Digital Equipment, and others—most are not willing or able to invest the resources necessary to become truly sophisticated purchasers in a now much more complex health care marketplace.

Multiemployer coalitions also have the capacity to demand competition by reducing competition on risk-selection. Because insurers must, in most arrangements, offer their plans—at the same rates—to all members of the coalition, and because enrollment is generally handled by the coalition or its employers, insurers have little capacity to target or select lower-risk groups. As competition on risk-selection declines, competition on price and quality is likely to increase.

Purchasing coalitions also have the potential to demand more than competition on price; they can demand information that better enables them to assess the performance and value of MCOs and

Purchasing Coalitions: Varying Forms and Strategies

The Pacific Business Group on Health (PBGH) is a coalition of large businesses, mostly based Northern California. The PBGH has been particularly aggressive in the collection of performance and satisfaction data and in disseminating that data to participating employers and employees. Additionally, the group has undertaken unique contracts in which withholds from premiums paid are used to encourage providers to improve performance. The group negotiates with managed care plans on behalf of its members. Employers then choose which plans they wish to offer. The group reports premium reductions in 1994 and 1995 of between 5 percent and 10 percent (PBGH representative, interview, 1995).

delivery systems. As MCOs and delivery systems have consolidated and as levels of organization have increased, the internal potential and need to generate information on organization performance increases. As it has done so, employers—and especially employer coalitions—have begun to demand, in effect, that such potential be utilized and shared with them. While the movement is still, at best, in the "best practices" stage, leading employers have begun pressuring and sometimes requiring HMOs and delivery systems to submit performance-oriented data. Employers and employees can then compare and evaluate plans based on that data.

As part of such efforts, employers may also demand that participating MCOs and providers seek and achieve accreditation or participate in national data collection and performance evaluation efforts—mostly through the National Council of Quality Assurance's Health Plan Employer Data Information Set (HEDIS) project. Employer coalitions have also been increasingly aggressive in distributing performance and consumer satisfaction-related information, thus improving the capacity for employers and consumers to select MCOs and delivery systems on value.

The "quality movement," of course, might move forward without purchasing cooperatives. But it may be that the information generated renders the cooperative, or some alternative to it, a critically needed component of future purchasing power. As (or if) choice for individual plan performance, however imprecise, becomes more available, individuals will need more assistance in making health plan choices. And they will want that assistance to come from impartial sources, accountable to them—not to their employers or to insurers. The cooperative is one means of securing that accountability. Table 8.2 is an example of this type of information distribution.

Some employer coalitions—led originally by public employee pools in Minnesota and California—are also fostering competition (on price and quality) by adopting cost-conscious-consumer strategies. In this approach, the employer (either individually or through a coalition pool) contributes a fixed dollar amount, leaving employees—who choose their own plans from an array of choices—paying more when they select higher-cost plans. Such cost consciousness, of course, has been notoriously absent in health care, as individuals see their employer paying the premiums and their insurer paying the bills.

Many believe that, in addition to improving consumer cost consciousness and thus increasing pressure on MCOs to compete on price, the individual-choice—as compared with the employer-choice—approach can increase competition on quality as well. Especially if given usable information on plan performance, and especially in the small-employer market, where employers may be particularly price sensitive, the individual consumer may be more likely than the employer to select plans based on quality. The individual-choice element available in a pool may have a particular value to small employers, who, for obvious reasons, offer their employees very little choice. Today, the vast majority of small employers offer their employees no choice of plan. Moreover, in part because they offer no choice of plans, small employers are far more likely to offer indemnity plans, which give their employees maximum choice of physician. The result is the offering of a more expensive plan, often to lower-wage employees.

In part for these reasons, penetration of managed care plans in the small-group market has lagged well behind penetration in larger-group markets. Yet, as an employer survey by the William M. Mercer company revealed, where employers offer choice, higher percentages of employees enroll in managed care plans ("Mid-Sized Firms Embrace MCOs," 1995). In all likelihood, then,

Table 8.2. Bay Area Business Group on Health:
1994 HMO Consumer Satisfaction Report Card.

California Health Plan	*Overall Consumer Satisfaction With . . .*			
	The Health Plan	*Doctor Seen Most Frequently*	*Care Received at Hospital*	*Plan's Health Improvement Programs*
Health Maintenance Organization (HMO)				
Aetna HMO	C	B	A	B
Blue Shield	B	B	C	B
CIGNA	B	B	B	B
California Care	B	B	C–	C
FHP	C	B	B	B
Foundation	B	A	B	B
HP of Redwoods	A+	A	A	A
Health Net	B	B	B	B
Kaiser North	B	C	C	A
Kaiser South	B	C	B	A
Lifeguard	A	A	A	C
Maxicare	C	C	C	B
Omni	A	B	B	C
PacifiCare	C	C	B	B
QualMed	B	B	A	C
TakeCare	B	B	B	B
ValueCare	A	A	B	A
Point-of-Service (POS) Average	C–	C	C	C–
Preferred Provider Organization (PPO) Average	B	A	B	C

Source: Used with permission of Pacific Business Group on Health.

Effective Purchasing Coalition

The California Personnel Employee Retirement System (CalPERS) is perhaps the best-known of all employer purchasing cooperatives. CalPERS has moved consistently toward managed-competition strategies in which benefits are standardized, and employees are made to pay (and can recognize) the full cost of more expensive plans. The system services over one million government employees and dependents, offering a wide variety of managed care plans. In recent years, administrators have moved from passive to aggressive purchasing, bargaining with plans over price. CalPERS reported average price decreases of 2.5 percent in 1995.

---

a pooling arrangement that offered employees in small firms more choice would result in higher numbers of small-firm employees in lower cost, managed care plans. Whether, of course, direct savings went to the employer or the employee would depend on arrangements between them. It can safely be assumed that the greater the consumer cost-consciousness in the employer-employee contract,the greater would be the number of employees that choose managed care plans. Additionally, more consumer cost-consciousness would mean that more of the savings from such a choice would flow to the employee.

Finally, the coalition approach allows employers to perform critical roles in securing competition in the face of consolidation among MCOs and providers. Employer coalitions can, for example, take steps to ease market access for new players, providing them a low-cost and direct marketing route to potential enrollees. Employer coalitions can also, as in the Minnesota case, even force competition between parts of large organized systems, demanding to contract directly with delivery systems rather than with their parent insurers. Purchasers, in this sense, can even foster competition between MCOs and providers, a value not lost on those concerned about the big getting too big.

The capacity of employers to promote a competitive environment may take on particular significance should employers extend efforts to promote direct contracting. As noted previously, some observers suggest that MCOs, in efforts to prevent delivery systems from emerging as direct competitors, may threaten those systems with the loss of managed care contracts. If employers, then, wish to promote direct contracting or to encourage delivery systems to form their own HMOs, they may need to exert leverage over MCOs opposed to such new entry or relationships.

Enhanced Purchasing Power: Limits and Threats

Enhanced levels of competition between MCOs and emerging ODSs, and enhanced purchasing sophistication and leverage in the hands of employers, offer hope that value can be raised by lowering price. But there is no inevitability here; a number of major caveats stand out.

Above all, any increase in value via declining price may be a relative rather than an absolute phenomenon. As discussed earlier, it is highly likely that advances in medical capability (including development of new technologies) and aging of the population will do more to raise prices than competition and increased purchaser sophistication will do to reduce them.

More important for our market focus here is that aggressive, sophisticated purchasing remains in the benchmark stage. Most anecdotal reports suggest that the great majority of purchasing coalitions still function more like price-takers than aggressive purchasers. Moreover, while they may be benefiting from increased competition among MCOs, most purchasing coalitions focus primarily on reducing their short-term health care outlays rather than on investing in strategies designed to produce higher levels of competition or quality. Whether, over time, the coalitions will prove a match for MCOs and providers—who are consolidating at a much greater pace, and who see whole businesses (and not just a part of business costs) at stake—remains an open question.

Additionally, as we shall see later in this chapter, data collection and performance evaluation efforts spearheaded by large employers and accrediting agencies also remain in the developmental stages. While most observers believe such capabilities will improve with time, a variety of factors, including market trends toward contractual arrangements, could complicate and inhibit the capacity to evaluate and compare both insurers and providers.

The Small-Employer Problem

Above all, there remains the ongoing problems of the small-employer and individual marketplace. While purchasing coalitions appear to be proving successful in lowering premiums, most coalitions consist of large employers (very few small employers participate in these coalitions). And many analysts voice concern that reductions in premiums to large purchasers may result in cost shifts to small groups and individual purchasers. That most large-employer coalitions show little inclination to invite small employers to join may suggest their awareness that reducing health care premiums is sometimes a zero-sum game, with gains for one being losses for another.

Surveys of employer health care spending clearly indicate that small employers (relative to larger employers) have derived fewer benefits from the new competition. Employee benefit costs for large employers may be stable, or even going down. But until 1995, at least, costs for small employers have continued to rise at twice the rate of inflation. Moreover, the vast majority of small employers continue to purchase relatively high-cost indemnity plans. As noted earlier, even in the new age of lower-cost managed care plans, 60 percent of small employers offer their employees an indemnity plan, and that's the only choice they get (Physician Payment Review Commission, 1995).

There would appear to be a number of reasons for the slow penetration of lower-cost managed care plans in the small-employer market. In a worst-case scenario, premium reduction gains being won by large employers may be yielding cost shifts onto the small-employer and individual markets. The ultimate result in that scenario is higher premiums in those markets, and increases in the numbers of the uninsured. In most states, few protections are in place to guard against such a scenario.

Theoretically, small employers could form their own purchasing coalitions. Their numbers, certainly, would suggest a daunting capacity to do. In almost any market, employers purchasing insurance for fewer than a hundred employees (or even those with fewer than fifty) constitute more than enough market share to rank as formidable purchasers.

But here a combination of business and insurance realities intervene. Few small employers have the time or resources (energy, capacity, personnel) to organize or even participate in coalition-type activity. Even more important, perhaps, is the susceptibility of the small-group market—including the coalitions it might form—to insurer risk-selection strategies. Some small employers may find attractive and (relatively speaking) low-cost options (at least over the short term); others are left with near unaffordable options, and there is little capacity to get all to see a common interest.

For these reasons, it has become increasingly apparent that addressing purchasing problems in the small-employer and individual marketplace, and especially the effort to establish small-group pooling arrangements, requires at least some level of government intervention.

Small-Group Pooling and the Need for Government Rules

Small-employer pools, like those operated by larger employers, offer member employers and their employees a variety of obvious advantages. Indeed, in many respects the advantages of pooling are far clearer in the case of the small employer. Such pools can offer economies of scale, reductions in administrative costs (much greater for small employers than for large), capacity to engage expertise in purchasing, and, most obviously, the enhanced leverage of greater numbers. Additionally, pools can expand the choices offered employees, and depending on how pools are structured, can enable employees to remain with the same insurer even as they change employers. In short, pooling arrangements offer small employers substantial opportunities to tap the benefits (and perhaps avoid some of the negative fallout) of the new competitive marketplace.

But such pools need not require any employer to join a health alliance type structure, or to purchase insurance through such a structure. Indeed, none of the twelve state-established pools formed to date imposes such requirements (Institute for Health Care Policy Solutions representative, interview, 1995). Small employers may purchase insurance plans through the pool, or outside the pool. In fact, some of the advantages of pooling—specifically, equal treatment by and access to insurers—can be achieved through a virtual pool in which the small-employer market is defined as a single pool, but for which no structure is created. (To be clear, such an approach, other than appearing less regulatory, offers no discernible advantages over creation of an actual pool that gives small employers the option of purchasing through the pool or outside of the pool.)

But, whether virtual or actual, the establishment of a viable small-employer pool requires the imposition by government of rules that protect the integrity of the pool. These rules must require that all insurers accept any individual or employer wishing to enroll in its plans, and must eliminate or at least severely limit the right of insurers to charge rates based on a group's health experience. Without such rules in place, lower-risk groups will be encouraged by lower rates to purchase outside the pool, leaving higher-risk groups with rising and often unaffordable rates.

To date, over forty states have enacted small-group insurance reform laws that at least move state laws in this direction. Some are weaker than others, allowing for considerable amounts of rating by health experience, and states wishing to encourage pooling will find it difficult to do so when the community rate in the pool is considerably higher than the experience rate some groups are offered outside the pool. Significantly, preliminary research on these laws has found that the movement toward community rating and the requirement that insurers accept all groups has not, as some feared, forced rates up (Jensen, 1995).

Institution of a small-group pool—virtual or actual—may also require government to establish rules on opting out of the pool. If, for example, multiple coalitions of small groups are allowed to form and self-insure outside the pool (and thus avoiding insurance reform rules), the pool could unravel, with lower-cost groups being enticed out and into self-insurance.

The same phenomena might occur if groups or individuals are allowed or encouraged to purchase medical savings accounts (MSAs), which generally enable individuals to purchase high deductible plans and, in effect, self-insure for a sizable portion of their coverage. Whatever their other benefits or liabilities, MSAs may have the effect of encouraging healthier and wealthier individuals to opt out of community pools purchasing standard HMO benefit plans. If such an exodus occurred at a high-enough rate—either by virtue of employers or individuals choosing the MSA

approach—the community purchasing pool could grow disproportionately high risk and low income. Even if the MSA itself is
purchased at a community rate (with all those purchasing MSAs
paying the same rate), the premiums for more standard plans
could be driven up as the pool of individuals purchasing those
plans became disproportionately higher risk.

Finally, and perhaps ironically, if an established actual pool is
to be allowed to use its larger numbers to demand lower prices
from competing insurers, the pool itself needs an exemption from
the state insurance reform laws. If, after all, insurers must offer all
small employers (even those choosing not to participate in the
pool) the same rates, the pool's ability to drive down premiums will
be constrained. (The fact that the pool is given such an advantage
does not, it should be emphasized, create any inequity. Any small
employer may join the pool and derive the benefit of whatever
reduced rates may be obtained.)

Government Facilitation of Pooling Arrangements

Federal or state policy makers who wish to establish or encourage
the establishment of pools—for small or large employers—should
consider a number of options.

• *Establish statewide or regional pools for small employers especially.*
The federal government could assist such an effort by furnishing
technical expertise (for example, risk-adjustment methodologies)
or modest start-up funding where necessary. The development of
risk-adjustment mechanisms that could protect MCOs and delivery systems that attract disproportionately high numbers of high-
cost enrollees must remain a particularly high priority. Without
such mechanisms, MCOs will have difficulty rejecting the inherent
appeal of strategies aimed at avoiding enrollment of high-risk individuals. Lack of a risk-adjustment methodology may also reduce
the willingness of MCOs to contract with those providers—for
example, academic medical centers—that may offer high quality,
but that also may attract high-risk enrollees.

• *Open state and federal public employee pools to other employers.* If
necessary, public employees could be treated as a separate rating
pool, with plans offering different community rates for public and
private employees. This would protect public employees against

Effective Purchasing Coalition

The Buyers Health Care Action Group (BHCAG) is a coalition of large Twin Cities employers known for leadership and creativity in, among other things, attempting to influence the regional health care marketplace. Over the past few years, the coalition has taken actions that have encouraged dramatic levels of consolidation among local health plans and providers. BHCAG has also supported efforts to enable employers and their employees to contract directly with delivery systems bypassing MCOs.

The Twin Cities effort may also be unique in that large-employer sponsors have opened the pool to small employers.

(In addition, another purchasing pool in Minnesota—this one purchasing insurance for state employees—was an innovator in cost-conscious purchasing. In 1985, the state switched to a policy of paying the full cost of the lowest-cost plan, with employees paying the difference if they choose a higher-cost plan.)

adverse selection effects, while still offering small employers an established bargaining agent with whom they might contract. (For example, the Clinton administration proposed in 1995 that small employers be allowed access to the Federal Employees Health Benefits Plan.)

• *Impose standardized data requirements for plans participating in government purchasing pools.* As will be discussed later, standardization is sorely needed here, lest MCOs be overburdened with data demands of multiple purchasers. Obviously, public-private employer cooperation here would be appropriate.

• *Explore means of encouraging large-employer cooperatives to accept small groups.* Mandating that they do so might be unacceptable politically. But such an arrangement is worth some creative thought.

• *Consider merging individuals into small-group pools.* MCOs might be allowed to charge a different community rate for individuals; but at least individuals might get the choice and leverage benefits of pooling.

> • *Consider legislation requiring noninsuring employers to offer employees access to government-sponsored small-group pools where they exist.* Such a requirement would be a minimum burden on employers and might ease access and price for participating employees. Risk selection issues would probably be minimal.

Issues and Strategies in Purchasing Pools

In developing pooling strategies, any government (and some private employers) organizing a pool must address certain issues. Most of these directly relate to how the pool can increase leverage vis a vis—or competition among—MCOs and providers.

One or Many Purchasing Pools

In an era of competition, the many-pool construct has a positive ring, allowing for maximum experimentation and for competition between pools, as well as between plans in them. But competition between pools or cooperatives would most likely occur on the basis of risk selection, with differences in prices in different pools reflecting differences in risk pools rather than differences in bargaining or other efficiencies. Addressing these potential inequities would require imposition of a variety of regulatory restraints.

Allowing multiple pools will also reduce the market share and leverage of each. This would be especially true if small-employer pools are limited to the under-fifty-employee market, reducing the total size of the small-group market.

Overall, the multiple pools approach may win politically. But the single pool appears the wiser choice and more potent tool, especially in the early going, when total pool enrollment may be limited.

Select Plans or Allow All to Compete

Coalitions may limit the number of competing plans offered to employers or employees. This strategy may maximize the leverage of the pool; acceptance of fewer plans means more enrollees per plan and thus, conceivably, more willingness of MCOs offering the plans to lower prices in order to achieve selection by the pool. On the other hand, such selection may limit choice. It may also be difficult for government-sponsored pools to deny plan entry.

Where the pool is large enough, both these strategies have potential to influence the competitive forces in a marketplace. Among other things, limiting numbers of plans accepted can produce consolidation among providers and MCOs. Opening access to all can ease market entry for new players.

Standardizing Benefits

Allowing multiple benefits packages, like multiple pools, can increase choice—but it can also complicate the ability of consumers to choose health plans based on price. Moreover, multiple benefits packages can reopen the door to MCO competition based on risk selection, as benefits can be adjusted so as to attract or not attract certain individuals (for example, by offering high deductibles likely to attract healthier individuals).

To date, most publicly sponsored pools have opted for standardization (Perrone and Manard, 1995), presumably seeing less value in a modest addition of variety and more value in clarity on price.

A viable compromise might define a number of benefits packages, with MCOs and delivery systems allowed to offer all or just one.

Employee Versus Employer Choice

Employee choice of plan, especially when a cost-conscious choice, can improve employee cost consciousness and ability to compare value, driving improvements in plan quality and service.

Employee choice may also have the virtue of easing new market entry for MCOs, perhaps reducing the tendency to oligopoly. Employers, by contrast, may be prone to pick larger plans with greater geographic coverage. Employee choice may also facilitate competition on quality, especially, as in Minnesota, where competition between delivery systems and not just between MCOs is envisioned.

Where employers wish to maintain the responsibility to select plans, a potential compromise may lie—at least with larger employers—in employee choice from plans selected by the employer, as practiced by the Pacific Business Group on Health.

Purchaser Coalitions, Evolving Markets, and the Future

The national body politic—and especially the business community—abhors mandates. Flying in the face of that reality, the Clinton administration's requirement that insurance be purchased through a health alliance was probably doomed from the beginning.

But as the marketplace evolves into a competition among larger and more organized systems increasingly capable of improving performance, the opportunity for purchasers to exert leverage and demand higher performance increases.

Out of this opportunity, it appears, the purchasing coalition is emerging as the demand side's best means of pushing suppliers to improve performance. The movement remains young, and many strategies are still being tested. But a review of the many new—and some older—undertakings suggests that purchasers, in coalition, may be moving toward the following strategies: greater use of alliance-type mechanisms in which several MCOs compete; standardized benefits; employee as opposed to employer choice; greater cost-consciousness in that employee choice; and greatly enhanced efforts to require competing MCOs to produce standardized data to be used by the coalition, by employers and by employees in evaluating performance.

Sound familiar? As discussed in Chapter Seven, what the Clinton administration had wrong was not the general strategy, or even in many cases the specifics of the strategy—but the requirement that it be implemented, and implemented in a particular way.

Beyond the Pool: Other Price-Related Public Policy Options

The establishment of purchasing pools, needless to say, is only one of several strategies purchasers can invoke in efforts to lower prices.

Direct Contracting

The rise of managed care and the ODS opens the door to direct contracting between employers and delivery systems. Without question, direct contracting offers major opportunities to increase competition among delivery systems and between those systems and MCOs. Direct contracting options may also offer the maximum in choice-oriented approaches: selection by individuals (not employers) of regional delivery systems (not organizers of those systems). Direct contracting, however, leads inevitably to a host of complex regulatory questions.

Some issues relating to direct contracting have already been discussed in Chapter Seven. Regulatory aspects of the direct contracting option are discussed in Chapter Nine.

Scope-of-Practice Laws

Central to managed care and ODS constructs is the concept of use of the most appropriate, cost-effective provider and setting. As organizations seek new configurations of providers, opportunities may expand to make greater and more flexible use of health care professionals, especially nonphysicians. Yet state law books are filled with licensing and other requirements that limit an organization's options to, for example, use a nurse anesthetist rather than an anesthesiologist. Rules pertaining to who can be reimbursed for providing a given service complicate the issue.

Clearly some such laws are appropriate and geared to protect quality. However, many have resulted from turf fights among health care professionals focused on who has the right to do what and under what circumstances. Where inappropriate or unnecessary for quality protection, these laws do little but stifle innovation and drive up costs for all. Unfortunately, those familiar with state legislative politics are painfully aware that such turf wars are intense and their results not easily overturned. When it comes to efforts to do so, "easier said than done" is an understatement.

Malpractice Reform

Mere mention of these words runs risks. There are few issues on which passions are as intense.

But the malpractice issue is one both of quality and cost. The fear of lawsuits—legitimate or not—may increase attention to quality, perhaps especially in capitated arrangements where physicians may have incentives to reduce referrals and procedures. On the other hand, as physicians are quick to assert, fear of lawsuits can raise costs, as physicians resort to defensive medicine and the increased utilization it engenders.

An analysis of these views is beyond our scope here. But current marketplace developments may make some options more attractive. First, the rise of managed care and capitation, and the anticipated rise of the ODS, may render the notion of enterprise liability both more appropriate and more acceptable. Under this arrangement, the organization responsible for care delivery assumes liability, rather than the individual provider.

Advocates outline several advantages to such an arrangement. For one thing, in an era of capitation in which plans are offering incentives and pressuring providers to reduce utilization, it may be more appropriate for MCOs to assume the liability risks of such pressures and incentives. Additionally, enterprise liability may provide incentives for MCOs and ODSs carrying the liability to be more aggressive in such areas as quality assurance, physician selection and monitoring, and review of capitation-related incentives.

To date, admittedly, there is logic—but no empirical evidence—that enterprise liability will reduce costs or enhance quality of care. But state or federal government-encouraged demonstration projects featuring enterprise liability might prove helpful.

Aside from enterprise liability, government might consider two other malpractice-related policy options. First, as a means of raising funds for quality-related research, government could require that a percentage of punitive damage awards (the portion of a malpractice settlement mandated more to punish the offender than to compensate the victim) be directed to quality improvement research.

Second, the increasing development—by researchers and organized systems—of clinical practice guidelines may offer some means of reducing malpractice costs. To the extent such guidelines become widely accepted, physicians may find that practice in accordance with guidelines offers some protection in malpractice lawsuits. While research relating use of guidelines to overall litigation savings or malpractice premiums is inconclusive, the issue is certainly worth pursuing. One option, clearly, is to give guidelines special legal status that offers providers following them increased protection in malpractice litigation. A number of states, most notably Maine, are pursuing experiments of this nature.

Anti-Managed-Care Laws

Several such laws were reviewed in Chapter Seven, as potentially anticompetitive, in that they might (unnecessarily) restrict systems from undertaking innovative delivery system changes. Most of these, especially any-willing-provider laws (discussed in Chapter Nine), would also have the effect of raising HMO premiums. So, too, might so-called length-of-stay laws, already enacted in three states and being contemplated in many more and in Congress. Such proposals, generally mandating a minimum length of stay for obstetric delivery, have won widespread consumer and political support. But in spite of the anecdotes that fuel support for them, the available research appears to suggest that relatively rapid discharge is both safe and cost-effective when accompanied by appropriate posthospital care (Hellinger, 1995).

Obviously, policy makers need to address such legislation on a case-by-case basis. And clearly, political imperatives may at times override other compelling considerations. But as a general rule, government might begin analysis of such proposals with two assumptions. First, where research might help answer the question at issue, it might be a wise and cost-effective first step. Second, where the definition or imposition of new rules or requirements may be left to regulators, as opposed to being fixed in statute, a valuable level of flexibility might be maintained.

Purchasing in the Medicare Program

Government policy makers also need to address purchasing issues in the Medicare program. While many (although not all) assume managed care has a capacity to save government substantial costs in the Medicare program, managed care enrollment in Medicare (less than 10 percent of recipients) lags far behind enrollment in the private sector.

Proposals to increase the enrollment of Medicare recipients in managed care, however, are fraught with political and technical hurdles. All agree, for one thing, that if Medicare is to increase managed care enrollment it must adjust its payment methodologies. At present, Medicare HMOs are paid relative to traditional Medicare per capita costs in a region. Where those costs are high, as in Miami, generally reflecting less conservative physician practice patterns, Medicare HMOs receive higher payments, and Medicare HMO enrollment increases. By contrast, where per capita Medicare costs are low, as in Minneapolis (where they are

---

Effective Purchasing Coalition

The Central Florida Health Care Coalition (CFHCC) represents 108 member companies with more than 510,000 workers and dependents. Unlike CalPERS or Minnesota's large business coalition, which contract with MCOs, CFHCC has focused on demanding improved performance from providers. The coalition has targeted regional hospitals, demanding the institution of comprehensive data collection to enable improved analysis of cost and quality of care. The new data system, reportedly, resulted in significant changes in utilization and cost in major regional hospitals.

---

almost 40 percent less than Miami), Medicare HMO payments are low and enrollment of Medicare recipients in HMOs tends to be limited (Kralewski, 1995).

Medicare HMO payment rates are also complicated by the risk factor. Absent a risk-adjustment mechanism, HMOs that enroll lower-risk Medicare recipients can either produce government losses (because the plan gets paid too much) or significant market advantages over other HMOs that enroll a more average or higher-risk Medicare population.

Even if such technical adjustments were made, however, enrolling more individuals in managed care would still hold only limited potential for government savings. This is, in large part, because Medicare HMOs—paid a fixed price from the government—compete on benefits, not price. Thus, an HMO gets more enrollees not by lowering its price for the government Medicare benefits package, but by offering Medicare recipients more benefits—including those generally covered in so-called medigap policies, such as prescription drugs or lower co-payments. Clearly, this may be an attractive arrangement for recipients, but it provides no mechanism for the government to save money via price competition.

To seek such savings, the federal government could employ a managed competition purchasing strategy, offering seniors a choice of plans—including presumably, traditional Medicare—with government paying the full cost only for lower-priced plans. Seniors choosing higher-cost plans, including, presumably, traditional fee-for-service Medicare, would have to pay the difference out of their own pockets.

Such a proposition, however, is a political nonstarter. Fears would quickly arise, with good justification, that traditional fee-for-service Medicare would be priced out of the market and that seniors would be forced into HMOs.

An alternative and perhaps more palatable approach, especially if phased in over time, might be to modestly increase the Medicare benefits package—to include most or all of the benefits now offered in medigap policies—and then allow competition between MCOs based on price. Such an approach might require recipients to pay more for fee-for-service Medicare or higher-price HMO plans, but they would at least be guaranteed a more comprehensive benefits package. And competition in an exploding Medicare managed care market might save government money, even with a richer benefits package in place.

Aside from these structural issues, some analysts suggest that Medicare could learn more from, and take more advantage of, changes in the private marketplace. Above all, Medicare needs to become a more aggressive, more selective, and more demanding purchaser. It needs, specifically, to abandon its any-willing-provider approach, and replace it with selection (and rejection) of providers based on performance. Competitive procurement is central to assuring high-quality service and low cost, and it should be available to Medicare (Etheredge, 1995b).

Additionally, Medicare might consider—as should any purchasing pool—beefing up efforts to monitor disenrollment from managed care plans. Indications that HMOs are encouraging higher-cost individuals to leave must be addressed aggressively, with penalties including loss of contracts.

Improving Quality

The new marketplace, it has been argued, holds considerable potential to reduce the costs of delivering health care, especially if purchasers are able to take advantage of the new opportunities marketplace change may offer. Thus, the potential to raise value (V) by lowering price (P) is significant. Moreover, one can argue, while there are hurdles in the path of lowering P, they are not insurmountable. For the most part, there is good reason for purchasers—public and private employers and individual consumers—to try to surmount them. Thus there is good reason to hope that the potential can be actualized.

Some of the same logic holds true for efforts to raise quality *(Q)*. The potential for ODSs to improve coordination of care, select high-quality providers, improve information systems, and develop and enforce protocols and guidelines clearly increases the capacity to deliver higher quality. But as compared to delivering lower price, the probability that the potential for delivering higher quality will be actualized is significantly lower. The hurdles are much more substantial—the most obvious being price itself.

The Potential for Raising Quality: The Glass as Half Full

There is substantial reason to believe that current market trends of consolidation and integration of health care systems have the capacity, especially over time, to produce improvements in quality of care delivered. Few dispute, for example, that clinical integration—while admittedly the hardest form of integration to achieve—has enormous potential to improve coordination of care. Especially when compared to PPOs or fee-for-service plans, more highly integrated systems (including many HMOs and ODSs) invoke greater use of protocols and clinical guidelines, include higher levels of peer group interaction, have more sophisticated quality assurance and improvement programs, and engage in more extensive physician monitoring and ongoing education activities.

Additionally, larger and more integrated systems appear more willing to invest in clinical information systems. Indeed, without the achievement of some level of clinical integration (or hope thereof), and without a significant revenue base over which to spread costs, investment in such systems would appear unproductive or unaffordable. And while it is far from clear today that such investments are compelling in the marketplace, given that purchasers seem more focused on price than quality, improved capacities for coordinating care set benchmarks and generate information on best practices.

Additionally, evidence is accumulating that larger, more integrated systems are more advanced in collecting performance, outcomes, and other data sets. Over time especially, access to improved data on performance will increase the capacity of accreditors, state regulators, and purchasers to evaluate plan performance and quality. Less integrated systems, including PPOs, have little reason to collect such information; moreover, where a so-called delivery system is just a loose network, there really is no organization to evaluate. Thus, the growth of the ODS may offer more than the potential to improve quality; it may provide the opportunity to evaluate and compare systems on quality.

And while efforts of accreditation organizations to generate and collect data on plans have their limitations, as discussed later in this chapter, there is little question that progress is being made here, and that MCOs are taking accreditation processes seriously.

The consolidation of physicians into larger group practices is also widely viewed as a positive development. There is general consensus that group practices offer broader opportunities for promotion of activities associated with quality improvement, including peer group and specialty consultation, group learning and improvement, establishment and implementation of protocols and guidelines, and identification and correction of inappropriate or unnecessary utilization.

An increase in prominence of group practices, and especially of larger group practices, may also mitigate the impact of potentially inappropriate incentives emanating from capitation. With groups of physicians assuming responsibility for larger numbers of covered lives, risk pools are broadened and risk is spread less to the individual physician and more to the group. Capitating the group will still exert pressure on the group to control utilization, probably a positive effect, and such pressure may well influence individuals in the group. But the risk is spread over the group, not to each physician individually.

Market consolidation resulting in larger ODSs and MCOs may have similar and positive risk-related impacts, reducing incentives to engage in aggressive risk-selection activities. Which is hardly to suggest that MCOs will not be interested in minimizing the enrollment of higher-risk groups or individuals. But as enrollment moves from ten thousand to a hundred thousand or more, modest levels of adverse selection are of less concern. Pressures on risk-adjustment measures, which attempt to assess the risk levels of populations enrolled in different plans and then to adjust payment to those plans based on the risk of their enrolled populations, may also be reduced. Finally, the prominence of larger MCOs, each more capable of spreading risk, should enable states to be more aggressive in imposing guaranteed issue requirements and in moving further toward community rating. It should surprise no one, in this regard, that the greatest opposition to small-group insurance reform has generally come from smaller indemnity insurers who rely heavily on their ability to underwrite in the small-group market. Eliminating risk-selection should increase competition based on quality and price.

The rise of managed care, and even of capitation, while raising the possibility of inappropriate incentives, can also yield positive effects on quality of care. Both provide incentives for improved preventive care and consumer satisfaction surveys have indicated relatively high HMO ratings on this measure. Admittedly, the probability that individuals may change jobs or move can undermine these incentives, which suggests still another reason for employee rather than employer choice of health plan; under the former, a change of job is less likely to require a change of plan.

Obviously, passing considerable risk to individual providers can raise serious quality and conflict of interest issues. But most analysts suggest, and some research confirms, that truly dramatic examples of this type of arrangement are rare and probably decreasing. Capitation of individual physicians (as opposed to groups) for more than primary care services remains a rarely invoked strategy. As for other financial incentives—withholds, bonuses, and so on—research by the Mathematica group found these to be modest, with physicians facing maximum income fluctuations due to such incentives (increasingly likely to include measures of quality and consumer satisfaction) of "generally 20 percent or less" (Gold and others, 1995, p. 83).

Indeed, a case can be made that from a quality or consumer protection point of view, capitation represents a positive step from insurer control to provider control over access to care. Given that an ability to control costs must lie somewhere in the system, the question becomes, where should that be? If the provider is not going to be in control of costs and services, that role will fall to the insurer, and it is in that circumstance that consumers may face the most serious denials of care. Judging the issue purely on an

Effective Purchasing Coalition

The California Health Insurance Purchasing Cooperative (CHIPC) is a government-sponsored cooperative featuring standardized benefits, and open to all small employers of less than fifty employees. It is one of the few cooperatives addressing risk-adjustment issues—that is, adjusting payments to participating plans for the morbidity of the populations they enroll. As of the end of 1995, CHIPC had over 100,000 enrollees. It offers individual choice from a variety of competing managed care plans. Unlike most government-run cooperatives, which control how much the employer and employee will pay and for what, employers in this program can determine the proportions they and their employees will pay for the coverage provided.

anecdotal basis, the most serious consumer complaints of care denied appear to involve an insurer denying a service a physician was prepared to render. Capitation of the provider or delivery system removes the insurer from that picture.

Capitated physicians, of course, or the delivery systems of which they may be a part, may also deny care. But while providers may adopt techniques and strategies to reduce utilization, true undertreatment does not come naturally to most providers. Concerns for reputation, a patient-first training emphasis, fears of negative publicity associated with bad outcomes, and fears of malpractice lawsuits may all mitigate tendencies for physicians to reduce quality or underserve.

Finally, some analysts believe that when markets consolidate and when penetration by managed care plans increases there is at least an increasing probability that competition will shift from price to quality. This may result because in such mature markets, price differentials between competing plans are reduced, as no competitor is able to provide the same services at a substantially lower price. Competition may then shift to other factors, including quality—as long as raising quality does not substantially raise price. Were it to do so, evidence suggests that employers might reject the higher quality.

Pressures to Reduce Quality: The Glass as Half Empty

Unfortunately, many believe, the downward pressure on price could also create downward pressure on quality. As MCOs and providers strive to lower costs and prices, it is assumed, quality could suffer. In spite of the chorus of assurances on quality emanating from MCOs and employers (providers sometimes express different sentiments), concerns about the impact of current market changes on quality obviously need to be taken seriously.

Quality, Price, and the Employer

The central concern for quality care today is the reality that price rules. This is in part true because the increases in market share and power, attained by increasing MCO enrollment, are viewed as critical to marketplace posture. Smaller enrollment of a higher-paying clientele may not produce the economies of scale or market power necessary for success.

Price also rules because it can be defined, whereas quality remains hard to prove. Thus, investments of time, energy, capital, and other resources in reducing price are more likely to produce dividends than investments in quality. Investments in new information systems, for example, will be hard to justify because they do not promise immediate reductions in costs and do not in themselves produce demonstrably higher quality. Even if market share were not such a critical issue, high-price–high-quality might be a losing strategy because its weakness (high price) is evident to all, while its strength (high quality) is usually a source of debate. By the same logic, low-price–low-quality can be a successful posture, since the market price to be paid for the (unproven) low quality may be minimal.

Finally, price may rule because, all things considered, most employers—especially smaller employers—care more about price. Especially in the absence of quality measures, freedom to choose on price expands. Employee (as opposed to employer) choice of plan might increase pressures on plans to raise quality. But even this strategy is undermined by the limited capacity to demonstrate higher quality.

For all these reasons, many market observers are less than sanguine about the short-term future of quality as a marketable commodity, as least as compared to price. Most seem to conclude that high quality is not necessarily rewarded and low quality is not necessarily punished. Early assessments, for example, of Pennsylvania's efforts to track and report on hospital quality found that market share of those found to be performing particularly poorly or well was not significantly affected by the performance ratings (Governance Committee, 1994). And in a recent national survey of employers, while 60 percent ranked "clinical quality of care" as "extremely important," when it came to specific indices of that quality the numbers fell off considerably. As shown in Table 8.3, only 20 percent said National Council of Quality Assurance (NCQA) accreditation was extremely important, and only 8 percent said the ability to provide HEDIS reports was extremely important ("Cost, Not Quality . . . ," 1995). Finally, in its initial effort to assess market change, the Center for the Study of Health System Change reported that quality was not asserting a heavy impact in competition between plans, that the state of consumer information on quality was very limited, and that it was not at all clear that high quality would win over low quality (Ginsburg, 1995).

Ideally, of course, the capacity to lower price by reducing utilization, improving efficiency, or reaping advantages of excess capacity may moderate the price-quality conflict, enabling MCOs and providers to achieve price restraint without placing pressures on quality standards. Indeed, it should generally be presumed that reduced utilization that does not negatively impact quality represents quality improvement. Moreover, there are clearly circumstances in which lower costs and higher quality move in tandem—as with cost-effective preventive care or new drug therapies that reduce the need for more expensive interventions.

But circumstances where the industry can have its cake and eat it too are not unlimited. Lower utilization does not necessarily constitute a demonstration of higher quality. And while lower price and higher quality can overlap in some circumstances, in an efficient marketplace we can assume that competitors will all take advantage of such circumstances. Therefore, over time, improving quality relative to competitors is likely to raise price relative to those competitors.

Table 8.3. HMO Evaluation Criteria

Factor	Percent of Employers Rating Factor as "Extremely Important"
Access/geographic coverage	72
Current year cost/premiums	67
Clinical quality of care	60
Financial strength/stability	49
Member satisfaction	44
Reputation of network providers	40
Ease of doing business with plan	30
Historic cost trends	29
Physician credentialing requirements	28
Ability to improve health status	24
NCQA accreditation	20
Physician turnover	14
Prevention/wellness focus	13
Ability to provide HEDIS reports	8
Membership size	4
Workers compensation/ Time loss management capability	4

Source: "Purchasers Don't View . . . ," 1995.

And almost as certainly, we can assume that—especially in the absence of evidence that quality is suffering—competitive pressures for lower prices can jeopardize quality as well as choice and service. Presumably there is a floor to such a spiral. But it is hardly clear where that floor is, or how it might be identified. At minimum, it may be safe to say that, even if market forces might not lead to lower quality, it is far from clear that as currently constituted they will lead to higher quality.

Competition on quality may also suffer because quality is primarily dependent on provider performance whereas current data collection and dissemination efforts are focused primarily on the MCO. And because most MCOs are really networks of many providers and provider groups, quality-related data offered to purchasers by an MCO may actually reflect performance of providers no longer in the network or not actually servicing a particular group.

The solution to this dilemma, obviously, is the collection of provider group-specific data. However, such a requirement clearly complicates the data collection challenge. Moreover, MCOs may have little interest in increasing the ability of purchasers to evaluate providers independent of the MCOs with which they are contracting. Such an ability could quickly lead to more direct contracting between employers and providers and to a loss of leverage for MCOs.

Other Quality Concerns

Even if general concerns relating to capitation and managed care incentives may be exaggerated, a number of specific areas of concern stand out. The shifting of sizable risk—especially risk that entails services other than those individual providers or provider groups offer—is clearly a questionable practice. And research—anecdotal and systematic—has identified several vulnerable populations that may experience particular quality-related problems in managed care and capitated environments: the chronically ill (especially the mentally ill), and Medicaid enrollees. In one particularly striking assessment, one expert noted that capitation rates for mental health stood at $2 per member per month, one-sixth of the $12 PMPM average in fee-for-service systems (Governance Committee, 1994, p. 73). Under such circumstances, pressure for reductions in so-called unnecessary utilization can become severe, quickly bordering on serious underservice.

Even where managed care plans have no intention to underserve more vulnerable individuals, a lack of assertiveness on the part of such individuals could produce the same result. And because the numbers of such high-cost cases are relatively few, overall consumer satisfaction ratings are not likely to detect major problems of poor service to the neediest individuals.

Where, of course, underservice to the chronically ill may lead to higher costs—as with the asthma patient who due to poor primary or specialty care ends up in the hospital—underservice may be far less likely. Indeed, this is an argument for managed care plans that offer substantial incentives for cost-effective preventive care and case management of high-cost cases. But in other circumstances (for example, HIV disease and some mental illnesses) more care almost certainly means more cost.

Concerns about underservice and poor quality of care may be most common, and most legitimate, with regard to the Medicaid population. As outlined in Chapter One, dramatic expansions of Medicaid managed care are anticipated. Yet evidence of serious Medicaid managed care problems have arisen in many states, some of which—New York and California in particular—are noted for maintaining relatively substantial regulatory capacities. Whether most states maintain a regulatory capacity adequate to monitor quality in a rush to Medicaid managed care remains highly problematic.

Accreditation and the Evaluation of Quality

There is little question today regarding the need to improve quality measurement capabilities, encourage MCOs and provider organizations and institutions to seek accreditation, or increase dissemination of comparative information on quality to purchasers. There is even considerable agreement on both the progress being made and on the limitations and nature of today's efforts and tools.

Clearly progress is being made. Increasing numbers of plans, reportedly about 70 percent, are collecting at least some HEDIS data. HEDIS includes more than sixty performance measures covering quality, access to and satisfaction with care, membership and use of services, and finance and management. More employers and employer coalitions are increasing demands that MCOs or delivery systems with which they are contracting collect and submit such data. The sophistication and value of consumer report cards, while still primitive, is improving. MCOs are taking accreditation processes seriously, with many observers assuming that accreditation will, over time at least, prove to be a critical asset—and lack thereof a serious liability. Some are even advertising their success in achieving accreditation. And approval ratios in accreditation processes suggest that those processes may be rigorous enough to have increasing value. To date, approximately half the nation's MCOs have undergone the NCQA's accreditation process (with most others preparing to do so), and only one-third have achieved full three-year accreditation. A significant 14 percent have been denied even partial accreditation, with the rest receiving some form of partial accreditation (Gottlieb, 1996).

Overcoming Limitations

On the limitations side, virtually all observers are quick to note where current efforts fall short. Most HEDIS measures measure administrative performance, processes, or use of services, but not quality and not outcomes. Difficulties abound in adjusting data from MCOs for differences in patient population mix. Many plans—especially those employing less integrated systems—have limited capacity to collect data. The performance data generated are less than consumer friendly. And data submitted by MCOs needs to be independently audited.

Naturally enough, the progress being achieved and the awareness of hurdles to be surmounted yield varying perspectives on the processes and prospects of the movement to improve and evaluate quality. But, overall, there is considerable consensus here: slow progress is being made. As one commentator described the most recent efforts of the National Committee for Quality Assurance, "Like the Wright brothers' airplane, HEDIS 2.5 is both an important achievement and a primitive instrument" (Epstein, 1995b, p. 59).

Most likely, a number of different planes, of different shapes and levels of reliability, will begin to fly within five or ten years. The ability to measure and compare performance and even quality of MCOs and delivery systems will improve. As it does, purchasers will have greater—albeit always imperfect—capacity to judge value in the quality-price equation. Recalling that Value (V) = Quality (Q) / Price (P), today's quality problem is that increases in Q may go undefined and therefore have little impact on V. Worse yet, if they raise P without visibly raising Q, V will decline. In such a market, price will surely dominate.

However, as quality assessment measures improve, increases in Q will have greater likelihood of producing increases in V, and as a result investments in Q should have greater value. Unless, of course—and here is one place where the simplification inherent in the equation breaks down—those making the choice of system adjust the equation by assuming that above a certain level or floor, additional quality has no or only marginal value. With such an adjustment, increases in Q beyond that minimal level would produce virtually no impact or not be counted at all, and the incentive to improve quality beyond that level would be stifled. Which, of course, leads increasing numbers of policy analysts to suggest that consumers (and preferably cost-conscious consumers) rather than employers should have an expanded role in health care choices.

Data, Quality, and Contracts

Such optimism having been expressed regarding the long-term future of quality assessment, at least two caveats seem required. First the trend toward POS plans may compound data collection problems, especially if out-of-network usage is significant. Second, and far more important, trends toward contractual as opposed to ownership and single-system relationships may compound the already significant problem of providing consumers with data on the actual delivery system they may be purchasing. In the age of the ODS, what the purchaser really needs to know is not the quality rating of the HMO—in effect, the general contractor—offering the plan for sale, but the rating of the particular delivery system (medical group, PHO, or whatever) that will be in charge of care. Thus quality assessment systems may need to be provider-group specific.

Similar problems will emerge where the outcomes or performance of providers no longer in the network are included in data compiled by an MCO contracting with various delivery systems. For example, high quality ratings for coronary bypass surgery will have little meaning if the academic medical center that performed them is no longer in the network.

Quality Measurement: Limits and Hopes

Looking ahead ten or fifteen years, one can envision significantly increased capacity to measure quality of health care organizations and much wider dissemination of information quality-related, thus encouraging more competition on quality.

But quality-seeking market choices on health care may remain largely a subjective phenomena—just as is the case with choices of

Effective Purchasing Coalition

The National HMO Purchasing Coalition is the newest entrant in the purchasing cooperative field. It is a national coalition, founded by eight major employers. The coalition will represent about 600,000 individuals in twenty-seven regions and anticipates using its members to bargain with HMOs for discounts and quality standards. Significantly, the coalition is structured as a for-profit entity to be operated by a consulting firm, perhaps heralding the arrival of a new health care player: the for-profit organizer of purchasers ("Employers Forming National Coalition . . . ," 1995).

cars, appliances, stockbrokers, or so many other things, the performance of which can be, and often is, measured. Moreover, there is always the reality that biased information (advertising) consumers receive will overwhelm (in quantity at least) the information received from more neutral sources. Which is hardly to suggest, of course, that the task is hopeless, or that the bar should be set too low; only that we should be realistic about our ability to jump over it.

On the more optimistic side, it should be recognized that the main reason that making quality-based health plan choices seems so daunting today may not be the absence of comparative data, but a lack of experience. The number of individual consumers who have been choosing between different health insurance plans remains limited; and most of those haven't been doing it for very long. In ten or fifteen years, when millions more consumers have had the yearly experience of making such choices, the process may seem less daunting. We may then find that consumers—using new and improved information, word of mouth, subjective assessment, and personal experience—may do as good a job of purchasing a health plan as they do of purchasing anything else.

Public Policy and Quality

The foregoing analysis suggests a wide variety of quality-related issues to which public policy analysts must direct—and in most cases are already directing—their energies. Some of these issues have already been addressed in Chapter Seven. Others, especially those relating to consumer protection in an HMO and capitated environment, are addressed in Chapter Nine. Issues of quality in Medicaid are discussed in Chapter Ten. Several other quality-related policy issues are outlined below.

Data Collection and Improvement in Health Care Delivery

Many analysts note the opportunity for public-private sector cooperation on data collection and dissemination.

As has been discussed, encouraging competition based on quality will demand significant expansions in the capacity of purchasers—whether pools, employers or individuals—to compare insurers or providers on a wide array of parameters. But the prospect of multiple demands for data from purchasers is already of great concern to provider organizations. Thus, while there may be a natural marketplace fear of standardization of any kind, there is increasing receptivity to some level of standardization in the collection of data. The opportunities for—perhaps even the need for—public-private cooperation in this area are compelling.

A sizable role in government funding for health services research—both development of clinical guidelines and outcomes research—may also be required if progress is to be maximized in these areas. Theoretically, funding of this research could be undertaken by the private sector. However, the theory has several drawbacks. For one thing, systematic health services research can be very expensive, at least from the perspective of an individual company. Benefits of the research, even if leading to the implementation of guidelines that lower system costs—for example, the identification of cost-effective treatment of lower back pain—may not cover research costs, at least not in the near term. More importantly, research undertaken by private organizations is likely to remain proprietary, while the public would seem best served by the widest possible public dissemination.

Government-funded research in these areas, of course, need not and usually does not imply government-run research. But government does offer the simplest means of pooling resources to undertake research that clearly needs to remain in the public domain. Again, opportunities here for public-private partnerships abound.

Government as Purchaser

In a number of ways, government could invoke its leverage as a purchaser to support quality assurance efforts. For one thing, governments may impose data collection requirements on MCOs marketing plans to government employees. Government purchasers might also require MCOs competing in government pools to seek and eventually achieve accreditation from specified organizations. Information on accreditation status could be highlighted in system brochures. And while government-run systems may be hard-pressed to deny MCOs the opportunity to participate in government pools, some criteria—such as data collection and accreditation—could be imposed.

Where they chose to be more aggressive on quality issues, government employee purchasing cooperatives could impose demands that participating plans achieve definable quality goals. Incentive strategies of the type invoked, for example, by the Pacific Business Group on Health (which withholds payments unless plans achieve specified improvements) could also be implemented. In such ways, as they have already done, government-sponsored pools can serve critical benchmark roles.

Finally, the Medicare program might well benefit from more assertive purchasing strategies. Most specifically, as discussed earlier, the program might benefit if administrators were to be granted authority to select providers based on quantifiable measures of quality.

Managed Care, Capitation, and Quality

In spite of general public fears and assumptions—stemming largely from incentives invoked and restrictions on choice—there is a substantial body of evidence that managed care systems, on the whole, provide the same or better quality than traditional fee-for-service systems. Even the feared strategy of physician capitation—if applied in moderation—may have a positive impact on quality by placing clinical decision making more in the hands of physicians, and less in the hands of insurers and of sometimes distant insurance utilization review procedures.

Obviously, however, attention must be paid to those circumstances where risk-sharing incentives can lead to underservice. These issues are discussed primarily in Chapter Nine. But, clearly, government regulators may need to strengthen their ability to monitor care of vulnerable populations in capitated arrangements. The prospect of rapid expansion of Medicaid managed care enrollments is particularly troublesome in the absence of adequate quality assurance mechanisms. To address such issues, government regulators may want to focus attention on disenrollment from plans. And to the extent government publishes and offers its employees report cards on MCOs, consideration might be given to weighting these surveys toward those with greater health care needs. Finally, as will be discussed in Chapter Nine, where delivery systems are found to clearly wanting in quality or consumer service, government officials should be prepared to use market sanctions such as public exposure of wrongdoing or poor performance as well as regulatory sanctions.

Pools, Choice, and Quality

Establishment of state or regional pools, as discussed earlier in this chapter, can offer considerable advantages, especially for small employers. In terms of quality, such pools can facilitate the collection and dissemination of information comparing plan performance and quality.

Pools can also expand choice for consumers, especially those in small firms where choice is lacking today. And while the tendency and ability of individuals, as opposed to employers, to elevate quality factors in plan choice decisions remains uncertain, increasing numbers of observers and pool administrators are moving toward the consumer-choice option, in part due to quality considerations.

Direct Contracting

The ultimate in consumer choice, of course, might include the opportunity for the individual, through an employer or a purchasing pool, to personally select the local delivery system from which to receive care. This option has multiple regulatory complications, as discussed in Chapter Nine. But from the perspective of competition on quality, it offers some clearly unique advantages. Above all, in the absence of comparable performance or quality data, competition among local delivery systems might, at least, be based on regional reputation. As it moves in this direction, Minnesota may, once again, be the state to watch.

Competition, Regulation, and Consumer Protection

The rise of managed care and risk-sharing payment mechanisms and the emergence of ODSs featuring new relationships between sets of providers have raised a host of questions relating to traditional state consumer-protection responsibilities.

These questions can be distinguished from the broader issues of how to maintain or improve the overall quality of care delivered in managed care environments. The latter might be labeled (perhaps optimistically) *ceiling questions*. They focus on how to improve and enhance quality, and on how to raise standards. Thus the National Committee on Quality Assurance doesn't focus on minimum legal requirements. It sets goals and standards that are, presumably, above what the states will require for licensure.

Consumer protection, especially as imposed by governments, is more focused on the *floor*—that is, on what is legally acceptable. The market may define whether or not an enterprise may thrive, but the law defines what it must do—including what standards it must meet to function at all. Government consumer-protection efforts, then, while they may seek higher goals, aim to establish minimum (generally legal) standards and to provide means of guaranteeing that enterprises meet those standards.

Such a definition does not mean to imply that state regulators should content themselves with guaranteeing that minimum requirements are met. Nor should it imply that government consumer protection efforts should be restricted to legal and regulatory processes. As will be argued later, state regulators possess a number of nonregulatory means of reducing the probabilities of poor performance and increasing those of higher performance.

Indeed, one of the most effective means of sanctioning bad actors may be public embarrassment that hurts in the marketplace more than in the commissioner's office or courtroom.

In the emerging health care marketplace, four sets of issues relating to consumer protection stand out as deserving special attention of policy makers.

- *The regulation (or lack thereof) of delivery systems that are not licensed insurers but that are accepting increasing amounts of risk and thereby assuming insurance functions.* Closely related to these issues is the controversial subject of rules pertaining to direct contracting arrangements.
- *State regulations and laws relating to managed care, capitation, and minimum quality and to consumer rights standards in managed care environments.* These include some anti-managed-care proposals usually offered in the name of consumer protection.
- *Regulations, standards, and means of enforcing them in Medicaid managed care programs.* This issue deserves its own focus due to past problems, unique circumstances, and future anticipated increases in Medicaid managed care enrollment.
- *Political (as opposed to regulatory or statutory) means of protecting consumers.*

Regulation or Monitoring of New Delivery Systems

The emergence of new, vertically integrated delivery systems (large medical groups, multispecialty clinics, PHOs), the acceptance of broader, insurance-related functions by such systems, and the spread of capitation are combining to raise new and controversial issues for state regulators and policy makers.

Traditionally, state insurance regulation has focused on those delivery systems accepting risk—specifically insurers, including HMOs. It has not focused on delivery systems that, generally speaking, have not borne risk. With regard to those systems, regulation assumes the form of the licensing and credentialing of specific actors (such as physicians, nurses, hospitals, nursing homes) not on the system (medical group, PHO, multispecialty clinic) in which those actors may participate. And it certainly has not focused on those actors as bearers of risk.

Today, as we have seen, more of these unlicensed (at least as insurers) delivery systems are accepting risk, sometimes full risk. Additionally, they are accepting more responsibility for the quality of care delivered, and for other functions—utilization review, complaint adjudication, credentialing of providers—traditionally performed by licensed insurers or HMOs. As they assume these functions, the question of how states should monitor or regulate them grows more complicated.

Three issues in particular stand out.

- *To what extent is there a need to regulate or license new delivery systems such as PHOs, especially those bearing significant risk?*

- *Under what circumstances, if any, should these now-unregulated and unlicensed delivery systems be allowed to contract directly (bypassing the insurer) with self-insured and other employers for the delivery of health care services.* The potential advantages to such contracting—innovation, a focus on quality, increased competition between identifiable local systems, and so on—have already been noted. Here we focus on consumer protection concerns raised by such arrangements.

- *Given changing patterns in the locus of care, is there a need to focus more regulatory attention on market sectors now delivering more care?* These include sectors such as home health and outpatient surgical centers. As these sectors have not been our focus, they will be discussed only briefly.

Risk-Bearing Providers

As has been outlined, provider groups of all kinds (primary care practices, PHOs, multispecialty clinics, medical group networks, integrated delivery systems, and so on), are undertaking a wide variety of risk-sharing arrangements—including capitation for some or all of the services in a benefits package. As a result, it would appear that they are undertaking at least some element of an insurance function, which is generally regulated.

Clearly, this is particularly true when the contract is between a purchaser (typically an employer) and the delivery system—that is, when there is no licensed insurer involved. But it should be emphasized that even when an insurer is involved the passing of responsibility and risk to a provider group raises significant issues.

For one thing, as a result of enormous pressure to reduce costs and compete for managed care contracts, some capitated providers may encounter serious financial problems or find themselves under considerable pressure to inappropriately reduce utilization of both their own services and of the services of others, most likely specialists, over which they may exercise some control.

The inexperience of many providers with managed care and capitation (especially in the case of solo practitioners and small groups) including an inexperience in estimating per-member-per-month costs, underlies such concerns. Fearful of losing access to patients and revenues, some may contract with MCOs at pmpm rates at or below their costs. An absence of recording systems to enable providers to calculate amounts owed specialists as a result of referrals can compound the problem. So, too, can the prospect that the patients for whom they are capitated are a disproportionately high-risk group.

To date, research has not produced reliable information on the extent to which such concerns are justified, including the extent to which aggressive capitation arrangements can affect quality. But the dearth of such information is, of course, part of the problem. Moreover, most state regulators have virtually no means of tracking the capacity of various risk-sharing provider groups to deliver quality care or contracted services and payments.

In view of this absence of information, some caution is clearly warranted, especially when it comes to the most aggressive risk-sharing strategies. Such was the conclusion, for example, of the Advisory Board, a private think tank well-known for its aggressive advocacy of capitation strategies. Researchers concluded, "In the absence of the strongest measures for reviewing and ensuring clinical quality, medical groups and physician networks should forego the inarguable economic advantage that accrues with individual capitation" (Governance Committee, 1995, p. xv).

Business Versus Insurance Risk

Some would suggest that the level and nature of the risks being accepted by providers do not constitute a consumer-protection problem. The risks being assumed, it is asserted, are business risks rather than insurance risks. They may involve risks to time, personal services, and even income. But they do not threaten the capacity of the provider to deliver the promised product. If the provider group underestimates what is required to perform the contract, its members may work longer hours and perhaps make less profit. But there is little risk that they will not be capable of honoring the contract.

But where physicians or physician groups are at risk for paying others for services (as with a primary care group capitated for primary care and specialty services or a PHO that must pay a rehabilitation facility), risks may be financial (insurance risk) as well, and questions of ability to meet obligations may be valid.

Even where the risk would appear to be largely a business risk, financial capacity issues are relevant. For example, a PHO that underestimates utilization will have overall higher hospital costs, including payments to hospital employees, contractors, and so on. Most important of all, perhaps, is the reality that one potential solution to pressing financial circumstances (whether business or insurance related) may be decreases in services and quality.

The Regulation of Risk-Bearing Delivery Systems

Such concerns have led some to advocate more regulatory scrutiny of provider organizations even where a licensed insurer is involved in the contractual relationship. For example, the National Association of Insurance Commissioners (NAIC) has been working on a model regulation for what it calls *health plans,* which might apply to various forms of emerging delivery systems.

However, attempts to regulate or apply standards to wide varieties of delivery systems may entail herculean efforts far beyond the capacity of most regulatory agencies. At least to the extent that the issue is one of monitoring providers contracting with a licensed entity, the wiser approach may be to focus on the latter, requiring it to collect and provide appropriate information about its provider networks and its contractual relationships with them. Such information might focus on the insurer's means of ascertaining that quality standards are met, the extent of risk-sharing strategies invoked by the insurer or contracting provider systems, and the means by which the insurer ascertains that providers will not be exposed to excessive financial pressures.

Of course, where there is no licensed insurer involved, that is, where the contract may be between an employer and a delivery system, the issue is more complicated—and increasingly, more controversial.

Regulation and Politics

Risk-bearing in the health industry once appeared to be—and sometimes still assumes the form of—a complex web of state regulatory and ERISA-related issues that few can understand. However, it is fast becoming a major political battleground between on the one hand providers and self-insured employers interested in direct contracting and on the other hand licensed insurers (including HMOs) and insurance regulators intent on limiting the scope of such contracting.

The interests of the various players are fairly obvious. Providers sense an opportunity to bypass insurers, giving them greater opportunities for profit and growth, more market leverage, and greater direct access to purchasers—a market tool that up to now has been largely the province of insurers.

Self-insured employers see direct contracting as a means of reaping the advantages of HMO products and the new risk-sharing strategies, while still remaining self-insured and thus outside of state regulatory frameworks. Until now, they have not been able to combine these goals, largely because—while they have self-insured for fee-for-service and PPO products—HMO products (entailing as they do the acceptance of risk) have almost exclusively been sold through licensed insurers. Thus, many self-insured employers will offer both a self-insured PPO and one or more insured HMOs.

But to some self-insuring employers, the requirement to purchase an insured product limits the attractiveness of the HMO option. For one thing, it eliminates the employers' capacity to benefit from carrying risk and forces them to pay other entities to do what they would rather do themselves. Additionally, the purchase of an insured product brings with it a host of state (or sometimes federal) regulations by which the HMO must abide. There are many of these, as discussed in Chapter Seven. But the most critical may be the limitations imposed on experience rating. Thus, an employer of a relatively young and healthy workforce may be unable to derive as many insurance-related benefits when offering an insured plan as would be the case under a self-insured plan.

As for MCOs, their interests are equally plain. Should direct contracting go forward, they would be deprived of the obvious advantage that accrue to unique rights to sell products and unique access to the purchasers of those products. With those advantages could go considerable market share and power.

From the point of view of state insurance commissioners, the matter is one of—depending on one's level of political cynicism— protection of consumer interests or protection of regulatory turf and responsibility.

Definitions of Insurance and Risk Bearing

The central issue, from a legal and regulatory point of view at least, focuses on the nature of insurance and the circumstances under which providers should be defined as carrying risk and requiring licensure to do so. Two surveys conducted by the Group Health Association of America and Ernst & Young, revealed considerable consensus at what might be considered the two extremes of the debate. First, commissioners agreed that delivery systems contracting directly with employers and thus taking on the functions of insurers should be treated as such, even though the employer is self-insuring under ERISA.[1] Second, they agreed that there was considerably reduced need for state regulator intervention when a delivery system is accepting capitated payments from a licensed insurer.

But between the two poles of the risk spectrum, the surveys revealed sizable gray areas, including the circumstance in which a delivery system contracting with an employer accepts some but not full risk, or accepts full risk from a few but not many employers.

Overall, these surveys, supplemented by other sources, suggest that many state regulators are often unclear as to how to react to a particular circumstance, hesitant to act in the absence of specific

---

[1] This definition has not yet been tested in the courts. ERISA plans would be likely to assert that state regulators have no authority to regulate a relationship between an employer and a delivery system. Regulators would respond that ERISA does not preempt their authority to regulate insurers—and those who wish to function as insurers.

state legislation—which often doesn't exist or may not directly address the issues at hand—and, perhaps most significant of all, lacking in awareness of what kinds of relationships actually exist in the marketplaces they regulate (Carneal and Gallmetzer, 1995; Ernst & Young, 1994).

The surveys aroused interest. But the debate crystallized around a draft bulletin issued by the NAIC in August of 1995. In that bulletin, which would only have legal standing if individual state commissioners issued it on their authority, the NAIC appeared prepared to raise the stakes. The bulletin argued, "If a health care provider enters into an arrangement with an individual, employer or other group that results in the provider assuming all or part of the risk for health care expenses or service delivery, the provider is engaged in the business of insurance. Providers wishing to engage in the business of insurance must obtain the appropriate license" (Draft Bulletin, Aug. 10, 1995, NAIC).

To those elements of the provider and self-insured employer community most interested in the issue, the bulletin was a shot across the bows. Among other things, it has begun to generate a series of organizational legal opinions (often for internal circulation only) of how courts might view the various positions, especially those that might fall between the two poles of accepting full risk from many employers and accepting risk from an insurer.

The issue, interestingly, was also emerging in the 1995 Medicare debate. At the same time as the NAIC appeared interested in restricting the direct contracting option, Republicans in Congress appeared interested in opening it up. Throughout 1995, providers sought approval for integrated service networks (ISNs)—later to be termed provider service organizations (PSOs)—to deliver the Medicare benefits package without having to obtain an insurance license. The creative notion behind the plan was that while passing some risk (largely business risk) to physician networks, Medicare could, in effect, self-insure for the insurance portion of the risk. Not surprisingly, insurers vehemently objected to the prospect. The issue was still unresolved as this volume went to press.

Regulatory Approaches to Direct Contracting

Should state or federal policy makers wish to encourage or sanction the direct contracting option, they will need to establish a balance between the flexibility such contracting may generate and the risks to consumer protection that the absence of a licensed insurer may pose. A number of options can be envisioned.

• *Require licensure:* Delivery systems wishing to engage in direct contracting could be required to attain licenses as insurers or HMOs. This, of course, is only a theoretical option, as it would effectively bar direct contracting as it has been proposed.

• *Change licensure rules:* Insurance licensing requirements could be reduced, at least under some circumstances. It is possible to develop regulatory schemes that permit direct marketing by delivery systems under certain circumstances and rules.

• *Base capital requirements on risk:* Solvency and other requirements could be allowed to vary with different kinds and levels of risk. Delivery systems might, for example, be allowed to sign risk contracts covering services they themselves performed (business-type risks), but not for services for which they paid others (insurance risks).

Many find this idea attractive, but the regulatory complexities involved are considerable. Additionally, such a proposal, to be equitable, would have to consider adjusting downward the requirements now placed on many HMOs, which could legitimately argue that much of the risk they carry is business rather than insurance risk.

• *Require reinsurance:* A related approach might allow self-insuring employers to reinsure delivery systems with which they contract. In effect, the employer might be allowed to provide reinsurance for the insurance component as opposed to the business risk component. The delivery system would accept the business risk. The employer, as in the Medicare proposal outlined previously, would assume the insurance risk.

Under such an arrangement, the risk to consumers would be no greater than under a self-insured employer plan. But the issue could grow more complicated as a delivery system contracted with larger numbers of employers, thus pooling and accepting more risk. In such a case, it would become more difficult to judge where business risk stopped and insurance risk began.

• *Require accreditation as a quality check:* Delivery systems might be permitted to engage in limited kinds of direct contracting relationships provided they receive accreditation from specified organizations. If they consider this approach, however, regulators

Two Significant State Variations

As part of efforts to find a balance between the need for consumer protection on the one hand, and flexibility to explore direct contracting relationships on the other, Iowa and Minnesota have enacted new licensure structures that include less stringent regulatory requirements for delivery systems.

• *Minnesota:* Enacted to promote community-based integrated networks, the new Minnesota law will allow entities such as PHOs delivering capitated services to under fifty thousand individuals to be licensed under less stringent rules than networks enrolling larger numbers.

• *Iowa:* In an effort to promote integrated delivery systems, especially in rural areas, new Iowa regulations allow PHOs to bear risk without obtaining licensure as an insurer or HMO. Key to the formation of such systems is Iowa's decision to grant such rural systems state immunity from antitrust law. As in the Minnesota case, requirements for such entities are less stringent than requirements placed on insurers or HMOs (Ernst & Young, 1994).

should avoid the blank-check extreme. At minimum, states should set direct contracting standards and then allow accreditors to judge whether or not the standards are being met.

• *Limit the amount of direct contracting:* Finally, delivery systems could be allowed to contract directly with a limited number of employers, thus minimizing the risk assumed. The greater the number of employers with whom the delivery system contracts, the more the system is engaged in pooling risks, and the more imperative it becomes that insurance-type consumer protections be applied.

Whatever the tolerance of direct contracting anticipated, states may need to consider the effects of such contracting on larger insurance markets. In short, if more employers move to direct contracting—in part to gain the advantages of avoiding state insurance reform rules—the remaining pool of insured individuals could be undermined, as groups of relatively young and healthy employees move to self-insured, direct contracting options. To address this concern, states may find it necessary to limit direct contracting to employers of at least a certain size, thereby protecting the small-group market from adverse selection.

Policy and Political Solutions Versus Regulation

As the foregoing suggests, trying to balance the needs of consumer protection against the desire to achieve some of the benefits direct contracting may offer is no easy task. The simple reality is that direct contracting envisions cutting out a function—insurance—that is a necessary component of the product being offered.

In the absence of viable, creative solutions to the direct contracting problem, two types of marketing arrangements may grow in prominence. In one, larger delivery systems (PHOs, hospital-based systems, large multispecialty clinics) may obtain licenses to market managed care products. In the other, licensed MCOs may market, among other products, specifically identified delivery systems. Employers could then, in choosing their insurance product, choose between the specific delivery systems the insurer offered. Some insurers might offer the same delivery systems, in which case the employer could shop around. In other cases, the insurer and the delivery system might be exclusively linked.

Undoubtedly, in such a marketplace, delivery systems and insurers would soon be fighting (as many are today) over who should get how much of the pie. Delivery systems, asserting that they are carrying risk, may demand that the amount of the premium dollar assigned to insurance risk should go to them, rather than to the insurer. But that would be for them to settle.

What cannot be left to the market, and should not be left to regulators and courts, are the larger issues underlying the direct contracting debate. Undoubtedly, all concerned parties will prepare for suits on insurance regulation and ERISA. But while some technical issues can be left to courts and regulators, the larger issues involved must be addressed by policy makers. The possible effects of various approaches to the issue—on risk pools, prices to be paid by self-insured and insuring employers, consumer protection, and the nature of competition in the industry—are simply too great, too value-laden, and too interconnected to leave to those debating regulatory or statutory definitions.

Consumer Protection in Managed Care

As noted at the outset of this chapter, insurance has always been, relatively speaking, a heavily regulated business. This results largely from the need to guarantee that the insurer will have the financial capacity to perform as promised, including the possible payment of very large amounts in a distant future.

Heavy regulation also results from the inherent interest of the insurer in paying as little as possible. In the managed care context, and especially in the HMO context, these circumstances can be compounded by the clear and direct relationship between providing less service and making more profit.

Which is not to suggest, of course, the existence of an inherent conceptual flaw. Clearly, incentives to reduce utilization can lead to lower health care costs that—depending on the strength and demands of purchasers—may flow largely to consumers in the form of lower prices. Additionally, as noted earlier, most studies have concluded that managed care incentives, including those encouraging lower utilization, have not led to lower quality, and may, in many cases, actually improve quality—defined, if nothing else, as less inappropriate utilization.

Regulation of HMOs

Still, the incentive structure inherent in the managed care construct produces potential for abuse that demands at least some level of, and perhaps some unique approach to, regulatory oversight. The problem, as always in consumer protection, is defining the appropriate level of regulation. Beyond the establishment of minimal protections, a balance must be sought between the value of additional rights for consumers and the administrative burdens and costs—as well as limits on innovation—that those rights might impose on the regulated. Viewed from a market perspective, the question may be posed as: Which consumer needs require statutory protection, and which can be left to the marketplace?

State laws regulating HMOs address many of the same issues. These include: quality of care and information about it; access to care, including such things as geographic coverage and adequate access to specialists; grievance procedures, including rules on denial of care and circumstances that may require immediate action; and distribution of information to consumers, including marketing rules, information on benefits, and consumer rights.

But the nature of HMO regulation in each of these areas varies widely across states. Some states, including many of those with higher levels of managed care penetration (Minnesota, California, Arizona, Oregon, and Maryland) have noticeably stronger consumer protection laws in place. Minnesota, according to the most recent comprehensive report on state HMO regulation, has the strongest regulatory protections, at least from the consumer point of view (Dallek, Jimenez, and Schwartz, 1995). In other states, often those with lower levels of managed care penetration but still some with high levels (such as Massachusetts), those protections are markedly less substantial. Indeed, the survey noted earlier found that most states "do not provide adequate protections for HMO enrollees" (Dallek, Jimenez, and Schwartz, 1995). According to this study, particular shortcomings were noted in the areas of access to care, quality assurance, information on quality that is available to consumers, and grievance procedures.

A full review of consumer protection rules in the states is beyond our scope here. Our focus remains on the potential policy impact of recent market changes. But policy makers may wish to consider—in some cases they may be compelled to consider—some of the following realities and opportunities.

Quality and Data Collection

There are increasing and considerable opportunities for productive data collection activities that would serve multiple interests—regulators, MCOs, providers, and purchasers. Collaborative efforts between states, between the states and the federal government, and between governments and independent accrediting agencies might all yield more consensus on what data should be collected, by whom, and for what purposes. Such data can involve questions of service (waiting times, geographic coverage, and so on), performance (such as immunization rates), outcomes and health status, consumer satisfaction, and even internal plan procedures (such as referral mechanisms and levels of risk passed to providers). Particularly valuable and relevant in an age of rising managed care and capitation might be means of identifying underservice.

Among other things, improved data collection could offer regulators more capacity to achieve consumer-protection goals by greater reliance on outcomes and performance of HMOs, and less on what are often more intrusive specific rules defining procedures HMOs must employ. Some of these issues have already been addressed in Chapter Eight. The point here is only that regulators may find their needs for quality monitoring and consumer protection functions well served by the enhancement of data collection methodologies and coordination.

Grievance Procedures and Disenrollment Patterns

State rules vary widely here. Twenty states require HMOs to provide written disclosure of grievance procedures, but most do not; twenty-one specify a time frame within which differences must be resolved, but most do not. Only six states require HMOs to establish a system of expedited appeal for denials of urgent care (Dallek, Jimenez, and Schwartz, 1995).

Admittedly, such rules can be burdensome, especially given overall findings that quality of care in HMOs is equal to that of quality in indemnity plans. But given particular concerns regarding the care of the chronically ill, incentives in HMOs to avoid high-cost procedures, and the high risks that can be associated with denial of care, erring on the side of too much regulation may be justified here.

Monitoring disenrollment from plans may also prove a particularly useful tool for regulators. Thirty-seven states, reportedly, require collection of at least some such data (Dallek, Jimenez, and Schwartz, 1995). Particularly critical would be information from consumers as to why they left a plan. Such information could alert regulators to circumstances in which MCOs were offering poor service or encouraging higher-risk individuals to disenroll and seek care elsewhere.

A focus on disenrollment and on those with higher levels of morbidity is also likely to produce a more meaningful picture of plan performance and consumer satisfaction levels than aggregate data on consumer satisfaction. While the latter can be valuable, and while the way the healthy view their plan is certainly relevant, the real measure of plan performance may lie in the perceptions of those who need plan services the most. Regulators, especially those with limited capacity to actively inspect plan operations, would be wise to put resources into collecting and reviewing data from high service users.

Disclosure Is Cheap

As compared to statutes and regulations mandating specific rules and activities, disclosure is a less onerous, less expensive and often highly effective means of bringing information to consumers and pressure on MCOs and providers. Information on such factors as consumer satisfaction, numbers of complaints received per thousand enrollees, percentages of individuals who disenrolled, existence of contracts with centers of excellence, rate of physician turnover in a plan, as well as what quality and utilization data may be available in a state can all be of considerable value, especially when widely circulated. Much of this type of information is now routinely collected by MCOs. Requiring that some or all of it be made public, and working with purchasers, accreditors or others to facilitate its distribution by consumer-friendly means (even including press releases comparing plan performance) would better inform consumers. At the same time—and just as important—it would increase pressure on HMOs to improve performance. In most cases, mandated collection of such information would be a minimal burden on plans.

Of course, where the licensed HMO is more a general contractor than a direct provider of services, collection and distribution of such data may be of more limited value. The purchaser or individual consumer will be more concerned with the performance of a particular medical group or network than with that of the general contractor. But there is nothing, certainly, that need deter purchasers of HMO products offered by general contractors from demanding more provider or network-specific data.

In fact, the tools of disclosure—and even some of the more aggressive tools of regulators—may, in fact, be more powerful in the hands of purchasers than regulators. The latter may feel constrained in demanding certain information—or may not possess appropriate statutory authority. Private purchasers have fewer restraints. Not only may they demand disclosure of data that government is unlikely to collect—on such factors as clinical outcomes and services, for example—they can also be more flexible and aggressive in demanding specific service and network arrangements. Demands might include increases in the size or geographic coverage of networks, the availability of POS options, or even limits on the amount of risk that may be passed by HMOs to individual providers. While these types of demands have been debated in legislatures as part of consumer protection packages, they may be more flexibly and effectively applied by purchasers.

Finding the balance, of course, between what must be demanded by regulators and what might be demanded (or requested) by purchasers may not be easy. Most notably, to be effective in making demands regarding consumer protection and related questions, purchasers need to know what to ask for, have enough clout to demand it, and care enough to do it. To date, only a few large purchasing cooperatives appear able and willing to meet such tests. Moreover, growing demands from multiple purchasers for different information can become undue burdens for providers and drive up costs.

Such logic points to the potential, noted earlier, for collaboration between private purchasers and government agencies. Collaborative efforts might determine highest-priority data needs, as well as the most cost-effective and flexible means of collecting and distributing information.

Disclosure and Capitation

The rise of capitation may present those responsible for consumer protection with a new set of questions: To what extent should consumers, or government on their behalf, demand to know how much risk is being passed to whom? At the present time, no state sets limits on the amount of financial risk that may be assumed by contracting providers. But several impose requirements on HMOs to inform regulators on risk-sharing arrangements or to consider possible effects of those arrangements on quality of care.

California, for example, requires HMO licensees to describe risk-sharing arrangements, and to demonstrate to regulators that medical decisions are not hindered by fiscal and administrative management. Nevada requires that an HMO's quality assurance methodology consider the effect on care and outcomes of arrangements that encourage or discourage use of physician services. Several other states—including Minnesota, Colorado, and Wisconsin—have similar provisions (Dallek, Jimenez, and Schwartz, 1995, p. 70).

But only one state, Arizona, requires HMOs to provide information to group purchasers on risk-sharing arrangements—including incentives or penalties encouraging providers to withhold services or referrals. The law, which took effect January 1, 1996, also requires employers to provide the information to employees.

As if to emphasize the conflict inherent in the issue, many HMOs impose significant limitations (referred to by providers and other critics as *gag orders*) on the ability of physicians to discuss treatment options or HMO reimbursement mechanisms with patients. Such restrictions may be instituted by HMOs to prevent physicians from recommending treatments that the HMO will not authorize. They may also reduce the probability that patients will learn about and object to being treated by capitated physicians with financial incentives to reduce referrals. Yet, clearly, such restrictions can both place physicians in ethical dilemmas and leave patients without information they may deem critical to their decision making about choice of plan or treatment.

Purchasers, of course, could demand such information. But most employers may have no interest in reminding employees of the means by which the plans they are purchasing may be lowering costs. This will be especially true as long as employees view the savings as going to the employer. Efforts to address this issue may thus require government intervention.

State Quality Assurance and the Locus of Care

Among the many changes in today's health care marketplace is enormous growth in sectors on which state regulatory and licensing activity has not traditionally focused. These include free-standing outpatient surgical providers, urgent care centers, and home health care provider systems.

Today, for example, most surgeries are performed on an outpatient basis, with the fastest-growing setting being free-standing centers not owned by hospitals (Frazier, 1994). And growth in home health care spending (including Medicare and Medicaid) has been over 20 percent a year since 1989, rising from less than $1 billion in 1989 to $24.5 billion in 1993 (Levitt and others, 1994).

As the locus of care delivery shifts, states may need to invest more regulatory resources in monitoring and assuring quality in these settings. One means of doing so is to allow accrediting organizations to fill the gap, with states making accreditation a substitute for licensure and oversight. But, as is the case with accreditation of providers seeking direct contracting opportunities, states need to be wary of signing off on consumer-protection responsibilities. At minimum, states need to define standards that must be achieved—leaving to accreditors only the task of determining if those standards have been met. Additionally, it should be noted, it is far from clear that accrediting agencies are up to the task. For example, only about one-fifth of the over 15,000 home health agencies are accredited by the Joint Commission on Accreditation of Healthcare Organizations (JCAHO).

Inappropriate Proposals

Many states have experienced highly visible and controversial debates over efforts to establish a variety of specific limitations on managed care procedures, including limitations on network formation, referrals, and risk sharing by providers. Proponents generally refer to these as consumer or patient protection. Opponents refer to them as anti-managed-care laws. Among the more widely debated of these laws are so-called any-willing-provider laws, which increase or guarantee physician rights to participate in networks; freedom-of-choice laws, which increase consumer opportunities to see out-of-network providers; laws that attempt to limit the amount of risk that may be passed to providers, especially individual providers or small groups; direct access laws, which provide enrollees access to certain classifications of specialists; and, most recently, length-of-stay laws, which attempt to guarantee minimum hospitalization periods, especially after childbirth.

Many of these may be well intentioned. Most seem either unnecessary or premature at best, and costly and inappropriate at worst. Not only may they increase costs—but, just as important, they may stifle innovation and competition.

More Appropriate Alternatives

In most cases, rather than enacting restrictive laws on managed care activity, one of three preferred strategies might be invoked.

First, research could be employed to determine the extent to which a perceived problem needs to be addressed (for example, the need to limit the level of risk that may be passed to providers). Second, state regulators could be authorized to collect information or impose requirements under general quality assurance mandates (as with minimum lengths of stay). Third, and most obvious, disclosure mechanisms could be invoked to inform consumers of issues and their choices regarding them (for example, the ease or difficulty of seeing physicians outside of a network).

Any-Willing-Provider Laws: A Special Case

The most prominent form of the anti-managed-care legislation, certainly, has been the any-willing-provider approach, now generally referred to, in its more moderate forms, as *patient protection* acts. By 1995, at least twenty-seven states had enacted legislation along these lines, although in the great majority of cases the legislation applies only to pharmacies, not all providers (Swartz and Brennan, 1996).

Opponents of any-willing-provider laws (including, it would appear, most policy analysts not employed by an interested party) maintain that such proposals lead to higher costs, render it more difficult for MCOs to coordinate care and implement protocols and guidelines and move toward higher levels of physician and system integration.

These policy arguments, when combined with the growth of POS options—giving consumers more choice to go out of network—and the political clout of a coalition of MCOs and employers, appear to be slowing the momentum of the any-willing-provider movement. Most 1995 efforts to enact such laws proved unsuccessful ("Doctors Are Losing . . . ," 1995).

Nevertheless, such network-related laws raise legitimate issues and concerns, the most compelling of which may be that of economic credentialing. HMOs may have incentives to employ selection screens or other means of rejecting or dropping (deselecting) physicians who attract—because of location, reputation, or expertise—higher-risk individuals. Such economic credentialing could penalize physicians caring for those with the greatest medical needs. An HMO, for example, may wish to improve its capacity to treat patients with HIV disease. It may even wish to do so aggressively and with compassion. But will it want to offer network privileges to physicians treating large numbers of patients with HIV disease, thereby attracting many high-cost individuals into the HMO?

During 1995, a rash of newspaper stories highlighted the reality that at least some physicians, especially specialists, were being dropped from networks. In some cases, the physicians charged that the cause for deselection was related to the patient-base they attracted. And increasingly, it seemed, deselection efforts were leading to lawsuits. However, stories suggesting that such deselection is commonplace and includes significant numbers of physicians may not accurately reflect reality. The research on provider networks conducted by Gold and colleagues, for example, suggests that both the numbers of physicians who get deselected from networks and the amount of economic credentialing currently invoked may be significantly less than some have feared (Gold and others, 1995).

Still, the incentive to avoid enrolling high-cost cases is compelling enough to suggest a need for compromise on this issue. That compromise might entail some procedural protections for physicians, at least when being dropped from networks, and an increased effort by state regulators to monitor (collecting new data if necessary) the extent of economic credentialing. If proven to be significant, additional regulatory or legislative action may be warranted, including a bar on the rejection of providers based on the costs of caring for the populations they serve. Overall, though, a focus on plan performance as opposed to restrictions on network organization may be the most appropriate tack. Thus plans may be expected to provide adequate levels of specialty care, employ nondiscrimination practices in physician selection and marketing, and abide by state insurance rules requiring acceptance of all individuals and groups applying for coverage.

States or the federal government could also address economic credentialing concerns by improving risk-adjustment technologies that could appropriately compensate MCOs or networks that enrolled disproportionate numbers of high-cost individuals.

Finally, in recognition of the new economic uncertainties facing physicians, all concerned might consider the merits of national rather than state licensure of physicians, or at least an expansion of reciprocal arrangements between states. State licensure serves little purpose for physicians—compared, for example, with attorneys, who may need to know differences in state laws. If physicians are going to face the probability of greater need to move from system to system and even state to state, consideration should be given to easing the regulatory demands of doing so.

National licensure might also help in promotion of quality measures—enabling plans and delivery systems to make greater use of out-of-state providers, most obviously those specializing in rare diseases.

Legal Restrictions: Protection or Problem?

State and federal policy makers may also need to consider how a number of statutes relating to managed care arrangements and tax status may affect trends toward integration and consolidation of delivery systems.

Stark Laws

Those concerned about laws that may restrain the growth of managed care or integrated systems frequently cite the so-called *Stark laws,* named after Congressman Pete Stark. These laws, enacted to protect consumers from inappropriate referrals or higher costs, impose restrictions on the capacity of physicians to refer patients to facilities in which they have an ownership interest. Stark One, passed in 1989 and put into effect in 1992, outlawed the referral of Medicare patients to clinical laboratories tied financially to the referring physician. Stark Two, passed in 1993 to be effective in 1995, significantly expanded the application of the law, making it applicable to Medicaid as well as Medicare patients and to referrals for an array of medical services, including home health services, inpatient and outpatient services, physical therapy, and radiology.

To many supporters of managed care and integrated delivery systems, these laws, even if well-intentioned, appear outdated, aimed at discouraging overutilization in fee-for-service systems. In an increasingly managed care universe, it is asserted, such rules may be less necessary. They may, in fact, stifle appropriate referrals between network or integrated system providers.

Critics acknowledge that the laws provide for some safe harbors in referral practices. However, they argue, many gray areas exist, leaving it unclear, for example, when referrals within a network would be acceptable. It also may be difficult, critics suggest, for physicians to take advantage of safe-harbor provisions. Most have a mix of business making it difficult to separate patients in terms of when referrals might or might not be allowable.

Still other concerns relate to the impact of the laws on the willingness of physicians to enter into some integrated arrangements. While the laws appear to suggest that both arm's-length behavior and full integration are acceptable, much of today's network-building activity—partnering, long-term contracting, and so on—is occurring in the middle ground between the two, where the impact of the Stark laws may remain less clear.

Finally, some advocates of vertically integrated systems have raised various technical reservations, asserting that the Stark laws, or at least possible interpretations of the Stark laws, may restrict efforts of systems to integrate physicians with other elements of the delivery system. For example, MCOs may wish to improve physician integration into larger systems by giving physicians equity in the organization. But such actions may then limit the ability of the organizations to own and operate labs, radiology centers, and hospitals.

Concerns about the Stark laws have been compounded by considerable confusion over how they would be interpreted. As of July 1995, there were still no Stark law regulations. The Health Care Financing Administration has issued a memo attempting to clarify some issues, but the effort has apparently done little to ease concerns of opponents (Terry, 1995).

Still, in spite of all the expressed concern about the lack of clarity, the potentially inhibiting impact on integration, and the costs of compliance, even most prointegration analysts appear to conclude that the Stark laws may offer some ongoing benefits and that what pitfalls and obstacles they pose for integrating systems are usually surmountable.

Thus, while such analysts advocate changes in the laws, few rank them as a front-line concern. Moreover, during the 1995 Medicare debate, even proponents of the Stark laws (including Stark himself) seemed to believe that at least some adjustments were necessary, and it seemed likely that some would be made.

Fraud and Abuse, Inurement, and Nonprofit Status Legislation

Hospitals, physicians, and other system actors interested in creating integrated structures must also consider the implications of fraud and abuse and various tax laws.

Among other things, fraud and abuse laws prohibit organizations, most commonly hospitals or hospital-funded PHOs or management service organizations, from paying physicians for referrals, which, presumably, should be based on patient needs rather than on financial arrangements between hospitals and physicians.

To prevent such payment, fraud and abuse laws generally limit the purchase of physician practices to fair market value. Paying more than fair market value can suggest that the physician is being paid not just for tangible assets of the practice, but for directing patients to the purchasing organization.

Similar issues affect the formation and structure of PHOs. Physicians may wish to have equal control over these organizations. But offering physicians more control than their financial contribution would justify could be defined as paying for referrals and, thus, as fraud and abuse violations.

For a nonprofit hospital, such transactions can be particularly complicated. If perceived as paying more than fair market value for a practice, the hospital can be charged with the transfer of public assets (a nonprofit hospital) to private individuals (physicians), violating rules on private inurement.

Clearly, such rules, however appropriate, can greatly complicate merger or acquisition activities, especially for nonprofit organizations. Which leads some analysts to emphasize that should integration activity prove more complicated for nonprofit organizations, such entities will be disadvantaged in the marketplace and may face pressures to convert to for-profit status. Such conversions could jeopardize, among other things, the system's overall willingness and ability to deliver charitable care.

A Special Concern: State Regulation and Medicaid Managed Care

One of the few certainties in the health care marketplace today is that the numbers of Medicaid-eligible individuals in managed care is soaring, and will continue to do so in the near future. Whatever the results of the 1995–1996 Medicaid debate in Congress—and whether states continue to enroll individuals in managed care via waivers in federal law or via state-run programs funded by federal block grants—virtually every state has embarked on a program to expand Medicaid managed care.

In 1983, just 3 percent of the Medicaid population, 750,000 individuals, were enrolled in managed care. By spring 1994, the number had soared to 8.1 million. And most of that growth has been very recent. Between 1993 and 1994 alone, Medicaid managed care enrollment grew from 4.8 million to 8.1 million, an increase of almost 70 percent (Rowland and others, 1994).

The numbers of Medicaid managed care enrollees was generally greater in states with higher percentages of non-Medicaid individuals in managed care. But, by 1994, the Medicaid managed care movement was virtually nationwide. While in 1991, 85 percent of Medicaid managed care enrollment was in just four states, by 1993, just 32 percent of that enrollment was in those four states. By 1994, only Wyoming, Nebraska, Alaska, Oklahoma, Vermont, and Connecticut were not using managed care in the Medicaid program (Rowland and others, 1994).

As great as this growth has been, however, there is every likelihood that the pace will continue well into the future. In spite of rapid recent growth, only 25 percent of Medicaid enrollees are in managed care today, leaving enormous room for growth. Most importantly, Medicaid is now the single fastest-growing program (18.4 percent of state budgets) in most states (Perrone and Manard, 1995). And while the evidence is hardly overwhelming (in fact, it's pretty modest), states are convinced that Medicaid managed care can save substantial amounts.

Overall, most of the growth of Medicaid managed care programs seems both inevitable and positive. But it also raises serious issues, especially with regard to the regulatory capacity of states to monitor quality of and access to care. Most states are largely inexperienced in regulating managed care plans, and especially inexperienced in regulating Medicaid managed care. At best, most have only modest capacity to monitor quality and consumer protection in Medicaid programs.

The same dearth of experience with Medicaid is true for many managed care plans, most of which have enrolled primarily middle-income populations. A Kaiser Family Foundation report suggests, for example, that only a few of the 340 plans now accepting Medicaid members are experienced at treating a poor, culturally diverse, and poorly educated population (Winslow, 1995). In the view of some analysts, the combination of state and provider inexperience, capitated payment structures, reduced expenditure levels, and the low income and education levels of the Medicaid population can create an environment in which underservice may be all too common.

The rate of increasing enrollment in Medicaid managed care programs is likely to compound the difficulties for states, plans, and individuals, as is the perceived pressure on states to reduce Medicaid expenditures. The same is true for issues of risk selection. While much of the Medicaid population is young and healthy and viewed by managed care plans as low-risk, some segments of the Medicaid population (even if the highest-cost individuals on SSI are not enrolled in managed care plans) can be very high cost, increasing incentives on MCOs to engage in aggressive risk selection activities.

Given these realities, it should come as no surprise that issues of poor oversight, abusive practices, and underservice have marred a number of efforts to expand Medicaid managed care programs. The early failures in California in the 1970s are legendary, but there is also more than ample evidence of poor quality and consumer abuse in current programs. Reports from a number of states—including New York, Tennessee, and Florida—point to serious quality assurance problems in marketing and delivery of managed care products.

In New York, for example, concerns about a lack of primary care providers, about plans enrolling more individuals than capacity should allow, and about high-pressure door-to-door marketing abuses have forced the state to undertake an aggressive plan to increase oversight of Medicaid managed care programs. An investigation by state health authorities of access to care at the state's eighteen largest managed care programs resulted in thirteen of the programs being cited for providing substandard care (Fisher and Fein, 1995). Included in the new regulatory scheme is a ban on door-to-door marketing and an array of other requirements and prohibitions.

Tennessee's highly publicized TennCare program has also generated a wide variety of serious complaints. Half the eligible recipients failed to choose a plan and were, as a result, assigned to one, leaving them unaware of what physician or hospital to visit. Hospitals found themselves faced with tens of millions in unpaid bills, as HMOs refused to pay for emergency room visits by individuals enrolled in HMOs that didn't have a contract with the hospital (Winslow, 1995).

None of which demonstrates an inherent flaw in Medicaid managed care, nor should expression of concerns be invoked to downgrade legitimate efforts of many to implement such programs. Overall, reviews of Medicaid managed care programs suggest that they can reduce costs (primarily in the full-risk HMO form), and that quality and access, if not improved over fee-for-service Medicaid programs, are at least no lower than in the traditional programs (Shortell and Hull, 1994; Rowland and others, 1994; Braid, Manard, and Carney, 1995).

But evidence from a number of states also suggests that adequate oversight of rapid increases in such programs may be beyond the regulatory capacity of many states, even states like New York where regulatory capacity is relatively substantial. The addition of pressing demands to reduce program expenditures may generate more stress than many state programs can safely absorb. It is well worth recalling that when California—a state with far more experience with managed care, including Medicaid managed care, than most—embarked on a major Medicaid managed care expansion in the early 1990s, the program director cautioned that savings should be viewed as a long-term rather than short-term goal.

These realities, if nothing else, suggest a need for caution in the implementation of Medicaid managed care programs. States may wish to give particular attention to marketing and enrollment practices, to means by which Medicaid recipients can be educated in the procedures of managed care, and to the treatment of particularly vulnerable populations. They may also need to review the capacity of networks and MCOs to absorb large numbers of Medicaid enrollees, and to develop means by which authorities can monitor quality and access. In addition, they would be wise to review (as we will in Chapter Ten) the impact on state safety nets of enrolling large numbers of individuals once served by safety net providers in private managed care plans. As a transition strategy, at least, states may wish to consider specific means—such as those being implemented in California—by which those providers get adequate opportunity to establish networks and bid for Medicaid contracts.

A Final Word: Consumer Protection— Publicity and Power

As suggested earlier, consumer protection is not just about regulation, complaint handling, lawsuits, or even statutes. It is also, in its most aggressive and sometimes most effective form, a highly public and sometimes even political endeavor.

Just as two hospitals planning to merge need an antitrust attorney, a good consumer protection program will need a publicist. Ultimately, consumer protection is not a one-at-a-time education process; it is a public process involving public education of large numbers.

There may be no substitute for tough enforcement. But enforcement should not be limited to legal sanctions. Sanctioning an MCO for refusing to provide appropriate treatment to an enrollee may be fine—but publicizing the failure to provide quality care is more likely to turn the imposition into consumer protection. Hiring consumer affairs officers to staff an 800 phone number and settle individual complaints about insurers is also fine (although very expensive and perhaps not the best use of resources). But compiling the statistics and holding a press conference identifying the insurers in the region with the highest numbers of legitimate complaints per thousand enrollees will have greater impact.

In the insurance business at least, the best education is public education. The most effective sanctions are likely to be public sanctions that educate consumers and thus offer the potential to affect an insurer in the marketplace. To be sure, such tactics must be employed cautiously, and often with appropriate caveats. But, especially given the limited resources of those charged with consumer protection, emphasis must be placed on means by which budgets can be used to educate large numbers.

If consumer protection requires education, it also requires power in the purchaser. Especially in a marketplace where competition rather than regulation is expected to rule, increasing the power of the purchaser must be the first tool of consumer protection. Means of strengthening purchasers—creation of pools, improved consumer information, insurance reform rules—have already been explored, and need not be reviewed here. But their value is worth restating in this context, and underscores the reality that consumer protection is a large-scale, not a one-at-a-time enterprise.

Chapter Ten

When Private Markets Fail
Ongoing Public Responsibilities

There is good reason to believe that—as least as compared to the recent past—the changing health care marketplace has a potential to produce lower health care costs and, over time, higher quality. The consolidation and integration of delivery systems, increased competition among MCOs, growing power of purchasers, greater focus on primary care and prevention, improvements in efficiency, reductions in unnecessary or inappropriate utilization of services, improvements in information systems and data collection and dissemination capacities, and a host of other developments all hold potential to produce greater value, including more choice than may sometimes appear to be the case for consumers.

To some extent, such a conclusion may apply to public responsibilities and programs, as well as private ones. Many of the same forces that hold potential for producing higher value in the private marketplace can have similar impact on public programs. Advances in the efficiency of delivery systems, for example, can help lower costs in the Medicare and Medicaid programs, just as they can in private insurance programs. Moreover, as consolidation and integration create larger private systems that may be increasingly focused on prevention and population-based care strategies, the potential for cooperation and partnership between private and public systems may expand.

But, overall, a review of public responsibilities and programs, especially safety-net-related programs, yields a picture that is somewhere between murky and bleak. For one thing, some developments in the private marketplace are creating grave strains on the public safety net, raising the most serious concerns about the economic viability of those providers that service the safety net, and about the capacity of the safety net to serve the growing numbers of the uninsured. Furthermore, in early 1996 efforts to achieve a balanced budget seemed likely to impose further stress on the safety net, largely be reducing Medicare and Medicaid spending, much of which supports safety net programs.

In this chapter, we explore how trends in private markets may interact with realities, needs, and opportunities in public programs. Specifically, we shall review the potential impact of marketplace changes on the safety net and the uninsured, on the Medicare and especially the Medicaid programs, and on the nation's academic medical centers and workforce needs. Finally, we shall review the policy issues relating to the growing prominence of for-profit health care systems.

The Fraying National Safety Net

For many years, the U.S. health care system has been marked by many indirect as well as direct subsidies for those unable to pay their share of medical costs and to those who provide services to them. But today, there is considerable political pressure to reduce spending on public programs, especially the Medicaid and Medicare programs, that provide both forms of subsidies. The rise of managed care, and the assessment (sometimes as much hope as assessment) of some that it can generate substantial savings in these programs, is a critical factor in this equation, enabling advocates of budget cuts to suggest that managed care can minimize or eliminate any negative impact of program cuts on program recipients.

At the same time, a variety of market forces may be exerting downward pressure on a number of indirect subsidy mechanisms, further increasing the economic vulnerability of those providers and public systems that have depended on direct and indirect subsidy programs.

The threat from government comes largely in the form of proposed reductions in Medicaid and Medicare spending. While the outcome of negotiations between Congress and the administration on the size of these reductions is unclear at this time, there is little doubt that these reductions will be considerable. Growth rates in both programs (now running about 10 percent a year) are likely to be slowed to somewhere between 5 and 7.5 percent a year. As a result, reductions in overall federal spending on the two programs are likely to total over $200 billion over the next five years. (Based on rough estimates of potential compromises.) State spending on Medicaid is also likely to decline, perhaps by as much as $60 billion between 1996 and 2000 (Holahan and Liska, 1995).

Whatever may be the effect of these reductions on the Medicare and Medicaid programs, their impact on safety net providers and care for the uninsured is almost certain to be dramatic, because safety net providers—public hospitals, community clinics, academic medical centers—are disproportionately dependent on these funds. In New York City, for example, the Health and Hospital Corporation, which runs eleven acute care hospitals and other facilities, receives 70 percent of its $3.8 billion annual revenues from the Medicaid program. The most extreme case of all—surely anecdotal evidence, but also perhaps indicative of the worst fears of those concerned about the safety net—is that of the Allegheny Valley School in Coraopolis, Pennsylvania, a suburb of Pittsburgh. The facility, one of the largest of its kind, provides residential care for seven hundred severely mentally retarded children. It receives 99.9 percent of its revenues from the Medicare and Medicaid programs (Noble, 1995).

In a word, the Medicaid and Medicare public insurance programs have indirectly subsidized the care of the uninsured and most vulnerable populations. However much providers have, over the years, complained about low payment rates in public programs, those programs—including the disproportionate share of their payments going to hospitals that treat particularly large numbers of poor patients—are the life's blood of many safety net providers, enabling them to treat the uninsured as well as those in the Medicare and Medicaid programs. According to some estimates, close to 25 percent of the total amount of Medicaid and Medicare cuts would come from reduced payments to acute care hospitals, with those having the highest percentages of elderly and poor patients, being most heavily impacted (Noble, 1995).

The anticipated movement of significantly greater numbers of Medicare and especially Medicaid recipients into private managed care plans, while perhaps a positive development, will further erode the financial base of the safety net providers, compounding reductions in federal and state spending with a loss of clientele to the private sector.

Theoretically, public hospitals and other safety net providers could seek contracts with MCOs enrolling Medicare or Medicaid recipients, or form their own plans and compete to serve those individuals. But many public providers are ill prepared to do so, and would be less than attractive partners to private MCOs. In addition to lack of experience in competing in private markets, most safety net facilities, long strapped for funding, have less sophisticated information systems and older equipment and facilities. The average age of public hospitals, for example, is twenty-seven years, compared to seven years for private hospitals (Andrulis and others, 1994). Additionally, safety net facilities are often located in inner cities where they serve large uninsured, high-cost populations, rendering them less attractive to MCOs. Safety net hospitals, it could be argued, might prove attractive to private plans enrolling Medicaid and Medicare patients accustomed to using their facilities. But this advantage is partially undermined by the general excess of hospital capacity, which makes hospitals serving larger numbers of privately insured patients much more aggressive in competing for patients in Medicare and Medicaid MCOs. Of course, the reform that would provide the greatest benefit to safety net hospitals would be universal coverage. With coverage extended to the uninsured, it might be anticipated, private MCOs might view public systems that had treated the uninsured (now to be insured) as more attractive partners and as sources of growth. But today, universal coverage seems a long way off.

Safety net providers are also less likely to be participants in emerging hospital-based delivery systems. Public hospitals are less likely than private (for-profit or nonprofit) hospitals to be part of emerging hospital-based delivery systems. While 60 percent of urban acute care hospitals are in some form of cluster, local system, or network, this is true only of 45 percent of public hospitals, and most of these are in looser networks (Roice Luke, interview, 1995).

To be sure, many safety net facilities are making substantial efforts to position themselves to compete in the new marketplace, by seeking managed care contracts of their own or entering a wide variety of partnering relationships with MCOs, plans, hospital systems, or multispecialty clinics. As we shall discuss later, this is particularly true of academic medical centers, many of which serve substantial numbers of the uninsured and are heavily dependent on Medicaid and Medicare funds.

But other examples abound. For example, San Mateo County in California has long run its own managed care network and competed with private plans. Boston City Hospital, reportedly, is planning to merge with Boston University Medical Center Hospital, and Parkland Memorial Hospital in Dallas has made efforts to supplement inpatient revenues by creating a network of dozens of clinics (Sack, 1995). At least one Catholic hospital, as reported earlier, has entered a joint venture with Columbia/HCA (Lutz, 1995). Many others have been consolidating facilities, reducing staff sizes, preparing to compete for state Medicaid managed care contracts (some of which, as in California, may be directed at public systems), and engaging in a wide array of other cost-cutting or revenue-boosting efforts. It is also true that various market trends, including consolidation of MCOs and delivery systems, are creating numerous opportunities for cooperation between public and private systems. (These will be discussed in the Conclusion.)

But while efforts of safety net providers to adjust to changing realities may be the rule rather than the exception, it is equally apparent that such efforts may often prove inadequate. The private marketplace may have only limited need of public providers. Anticipated reductions in government programs may be simply too severe. Growing pressure from higher numbers of the uninsured may be too great. As a result, it is increasingly common to hear projections of sizable numbers of closures (up to 40 percent of public hospitals over the next ten years) of public and other safety net hospitals.

Which is not to suggest that all the efforts of safety net providers, and, it should be added, their political supporters, are necessarily one and the same with the public interest. Nor is it to suggest that closures of some if not many safety net facilities would necessarily be unwise. Many agree that—especially given trends in hospital utilization—the nation has too many public hospitals, just as it has too many private hospitals. (There has been no such hospital closure in a major city since 1977.) And many argue that public systems would be wiser to spend their limited resources on community outpatient facilities, rather than struggling to maintain large inpatient operations. Many question, for example, recent decisions in financially strapped Los Angeles County to enact massive cuts in outpatient facilities and clinics while maintaining and even rebuilding inpatient capacity. Such health care questions frequently become political-economic issues featuring debates over jobs and masking the desire of public officials to maintain control over large health care budgets.

Still, the overall picture is clearly a bleak one. Stress is increasing on a frayed and fraying safety net that is almost certainly going to be required to do more with less.

Increasing competition in the private marketplace further complicates the safety net problem. In the now-disappearing world of fee-for-service and ever-rising premiums, many hospitals—public and private—were able to shift the cost of treating the uninsured to private payers. By one estimate, hospitals lost $26 billion in 1992 providing services to Medicaid and Medicare patients and to the uninsured, much of which they were able to recoup by raising prices to the privately insured (Shactman and Altman, 1995, citing Physician Payment Review Commission Report to Congress, 1994). But today, demands of employers for lower premium costs, and needs of providers to reduce costs to render themselves more attractive to networks, reduce the willingness and ability of providers to offer uncompensated care. Even before the dramatic increases in managed care penetration and competition during the 1990s, there was evidence of a reduction in the willingness of private hospitals (including nonprofits) to care for the uninsured. According to the National Public Health and Hospital Institute, between 1980 and 1990, the share of public hospital budgets that went to care for the uninsured increased by 17 percent while the share of private hospital budgets going to that purpose declined by 16 percent (Sack, 1995).

Hospitals that do wish to provide such care find they must charge paying clients more. Thus, their costs are higher, and their ability to compete for managed care contracts jeopardized. Particularly hard-hit by these forces are academic medical centers, which find their higher costs and their need to shift costs of treating uninsured and Medicaid patients leave them with serious liabilities in seeking to win contracts with MCOs.

Related to—and compounding—the cost-shift problem may be the rising influence of for-profit systems, especially for-profit hospital systems. This development will be discussed in more detail later. But should more nonprofit hospitals convert to for-profit status, or should more nonprofit hospitals find themselves linked to, and perhaps more dependent on, for-profit hospital chains, the capacity of the nation's delivery system to generate charity care may be further eroded.

The Uninsured: Still Growing in Numbers

To many economists, the decline of indirect subsidies in and of itself might be viewed as a positive development. Indirect subsidies, most would argue, create economic distortions and are inherently inefficient. But, obviously, for those concerned about the fabric of the safety net, indirect subsidies are preferable to no subsidies at all. And, at this time at least, it does not appear that direct subsidies are likely to be forthcoming.

To this reality must be added the most discouraging of ongoing trends: in the face of declining resources, the numbers of individuals the safety net needs to serve continue to grow. The uninsured population continues to climb by approximately 1.2 million a month. By the end of 1995, about 44 million individuals (18.7 percent of the under-sixty-five population) were uninsured, up from about 33 million in 1988 (Bradsher, 1995, citing Employee Benefit Research Institute). If current trends in employer-sponsored insurance continue, according to one expert, by 2002 the numbers of the uninsured could reach 55 million (Freudenheim, 1995a, quoting Steve Long of the RAND Corporation), about 17 million more than when the Clinton administration launched its effort to provide universal coverage in 1993.

Underlying these numbers is the assumption, questioned by few, that whatever reductions in premiums (or in rates of premium increase) marketplace change may foster will not lead to significant increases in employer-sponsored coverage. Nor can help be expected from small-group market reforms. These may be critically valuable in terms of enabling groups to keep insurance. And in the case of some employers with high-risk workforces, the limits on the imposition of experience rating may reduce premiums enough to make once-unaffordable coverage affordable. But, over-all, these reforms are not expected to lower premiums, and it is the cost of insurance that is the predominant reason that small employers do not provide insurance coverage (Morrisey, Jensen, and Morlock, 1994).

Thus, the numbers of the uninsured will almost certainly continue to rise, while the capacity of safety net mechanisms to care for them may shrink.

With the federal government (Congress, at least) apparently prepared to reduce efforts to support the uninsured, the burdens of doing so will fall to the states. Here there may be a least one bright spot. In a 1995 ruling, the Supreme Court appears to have opened the door to some state reform efforts aimed at aiding the indigent. Specifically, the Court ruled in a New York case that the state could impose surcharges on hospital bills paid by insurers and HMOs providing coverage to employee-benefit plans. The surcharges had been challenged as violating ERISA, which preempts state laws relating to employee benefit plans. The law has generally insulated employee benefit plans from state regulation, including state efforts to raise revenues from those plans to pay health costs of the indigent.

The new opportunity, of course, will only be as good as the willingness of states to take advantage of it. Many appear interested in doing so, with a number of states already having enacted rules similar to those in New York (Barrett, 1995).

Expanding Medicaid

An alternative means of addressing safety net issues and problems of the uninsured might lie in the expansion of Medicaid. The program has, in fact, been the nation's most prominent means of keeping the growing numbers of the uninsured, especially pregnant women and children, in check. Between 1988 and 1994, for example, the percentage of children under eighteen years of age who were covered by employer-based insurance fell from 66 percent to 59 percent. Over the same period, the numbers of children covered by the Medicaid program rose from 16 percent to 26 percent (Rich, 1995). Such Medicaid expansions were, not surprisingly, a large factor in Medicaid cost growth. Between 1992 and

1993, after various Congressional efforts to control expenditure growth, fully two-thirds of the increases in Medicaid expenditures resulted from increased enrollment (Koppelman, 1995).

Conceivably, if Medicaid managed care can reduce costs while assuring at least comparable quality to traditional Medicaid fee-for-service, the program would have the potential to continue to play such a backstop role. Here, according to research reviews, the evidence is mixed, in part due to considerable differences in Medicaid MCO designs. Overall, it remains clear that Medicaid managed care has not, certainly not with any consistency, achieved a number of fundamental goals relating to access and quality of care. While there is some evidence of improved access, there is also evidence that programs may be falling short of goals of increasing access to preventive and prenatal care, in part at least because of the high turnover among Medicaid enrollees (Rowland and others, 1994). And, overall, quality in Medicaid MCOs may be no higher (although apparently no lower either) than in fee-for-service Medicaid (Shortell and Hull, 1994; Rowland and others, 1994). Finally, to date, there is little evidence relating to outcomes (Braid, Maynard, and Carney, 1995).

But on the critical issue of cost, there is a growing body of evidence—anecdotal and systematic—that Medicaid managed care has some capacity to reduce costs. Researchers appear to differ on some issues—for example, whether inpatient utilization is lower in Medicaid MCOs than in Medicaid fee-for-service—and it may also be true that reductions in Medicaid costs are the results of cost shifts to the private sector. Still, reviews are suggesting that Medicaid managed care may be reducing costs, especially, perhaps, when care is delivered by prepaid capitated plans as opposed to other managed care models (Rowland and others, 1994).

The best news, in this regard, may come from the Arizona program, which appears to have produced substantial savings (as well as a slower rate of cost growth) over what the state would have spent on a traditional Medicaid program (Shortell and Hull, 1994). (Significantly, however, Arizona state officials warn that such savings may not come easily or quickly, and may require multimillion dollar investments in information systems needed in bargaining with providers over prices and in monitoring quality) (Neville, 1995). Overall, then, the research evidence appears to suggest that

Medicaid managed care may have some capacity to lower costs without lowering quality and service to recipients.

The marketplace, moreover, would appear to be exuding considerable confidence in such a conclusion, at least with regard to cost. Reports from across the country suggest that provider groups of all kinds are already competing or planning to compete for Medicaid managed care contracts. According to many analysts, such interest has a number of causes. Above all, many provider groups and MCOs believe they can make money on Medicaid managed care. Given reductions in premiums in some markets for employer-sponsored plans, Medicaid managed care premiums may appear more attractive than was once the case.

Even those less confident of the ability to make profits may see growth in numbers of covered lives (as discussed earlier) as central to long-term success. Even breaking even on Medicaid contracts can enhance an overall business posture, creating greater market share and leverage over providers and generating larger revenues, which may be attractive to investors.

Finally, some suggest that many MCOs serving the Medicaid population have found some concerns about that population to be unwarranted. Early fears about problems stemming from cultural diversity, language barriers, and treatment of low-income populations have often turned out to be unjustified. To be sure, enrollment of large numbers of Medicaid recipients may require a number of organizational adjustments. But, according to many reports, those adjustments are manageable.

One might thus anticipate and even hope that Medicaid managed care holds true potential for reducing program costs. If savings are appropriately directed, Medicaid could continue to offer some buffer to the problems of the expanding uninsured population and the fraying safety net.

However, political forces are such that only the first of these goals may be achieved, and even that achievement must be viewed as problematic. If overall program cuts are significant (for example, reducing Medicaid's rate of growth from about 10 percent a year to 5 percent), states may find that, at very best, they are only able to hold their own in covering those currently eligible for the program. At worst, eligibility rules will have to be tightened or benefits reduced.

For example, if the anticipated average annual Medicaid growth rate of 9.8 percent is capped at 5 percent for both the federal government and the states, total state and federal spending on the program (reductions would vary by state) in the year 2000 would be a full 20 percent below current projections (Holahan and Liska, 1995).

To these numbers must be added the reality that 70 percent of Medicaid spending is on the 25 percent of Medicaid recipients who are elderly or disabled, populations that have rarely been covered by MCOs (Braid, Maynard, and Carney, 1995). Thus, even if MCOs in the year 2000 were able to reduce spending levels for the remaining Medicaid population (mostly poor women and children) by as much as 15 percent (a high figure by any standard), states would still be far short of the overall 20 percent program savings that would be required. Such reductions would recover only about 4 or 5 percentage points, reducing the estimated shortfall to around 15 percent.

Projections developed by the state of Maryland offer one example of this predicament. An analysis developed by health policy consultants at the University of Maryland concluded that transferring two-thirds of all state Medicaid recipients (including those with chronic mental illness) into tightly controlled MCOs would produce less than half of the $2.8 million that Maryland would lose as a result of congressional proposals. The blueprint abandons the state goal of enrolling an additional hundred thousand people in the Medicaid program (Goldstein, 1995).

In short, it is very difficult—if not impossible–to imagine how managed care could produce anywhere near the savings required to allow Medicaid to continue serving the populations now eligible at similar levels of benefits. Whatever the potential of Medicaid managed care to ease the crisis of the uninsured, it appears unlikely that that potential will be tapped. Indeed, it must be considered far more likely that proposed reductions in Medicaid spending will more than offset any gains managed care might produce, leaving a significant net increase in the numbers of the uninsured, perhaps as many as five million (Koppelman, 1995; Freudenheim, 1995a).

Of course, many disagree with such discouraging scenarios, believing that substantially lower rates of growth in Medicaid need not lead to negative results for actual and potential Medicaid beneficiaries. Among the more interesting arguments put forward in this regard was one offered by Michigan's Medicaid director. He suggested that a capped federal allotment would enable (perhaps force) state legislators to bring more pressure on providers to increase delivery system efficiency and to consider closing hospitals—which, as we have seen, is a particularly sticky political task (Koppelman, 1995).

Such arguments, based in political reality, may have merit. However, they probably do not justify the extent of the reductions being considered, or the risks posed by those reductions.

Medicare, Managed Care, and the Safety Net

In some respects, the Medicare story is much the same as the Medicaid story. Medicare administrators and many policy analysts believe estimates of potential Medicare managed care savings are greatly exaggerated. But all observers anticipate rapid growth in Medicare MCOs, and most assume that (especially once payment formula problems are resolved) managed care can achieve significant savings in the Medicare program. Indeed, most believe that the potential savings in Medicare are substantially greater than in the Medicaid program. Medicare pays more for services than Medicaid, suggesting greater potential for lower costs. More importantly, Medicare has much higher per capita costs, such that 5 percent to 10 percent reductions in per capita payments produce considerably larger dollar savings.

But, as is the case with Medicaid, the capacity of managed care to reduce Medicare costs will do little to assist government in addressing its other health care responsibilities. Savings in Medicare—whether produced by lower provider payment rates or enrollment of more beneficiaries in managed care—appear earmarked for deficit reduction or other non-health-care purposes. Indeed, if anything, those reductions are likely to increase stress on the government-provided safety net by reducing the flow of funds to safety net providers. Increases in Medicare managed care may have the same effect, as public hospitals and academic medical centers lose Medicare patients to private MCOs.

Anticipated Medicare/Medicaid reductions may also generate a negative impact on employer-sponsored coverage, reducing spending in public programs may result in a cost shift to private payers. Should that cost shift be directed at weaker, smaller employers, the result could be decisions on the part of some employers to drop or reduce coverage. At least one estimate, offered by the research firm of Lewin-VHI, suggested that Medicare/Medicaid reductions approved by Congress in late 1995 (actual reductions will undoubtedly be significantly less) could produce a cost shift of over $90 to employers and individuals, increasing premiums by about $90 or 2 percent to 3 percent, and increasing the numbers of the uninsured by over 500,000 (Freudenheim, 1995b).

Which is not to suggest, certainly, that all the reforms being contemplated in the Medicare program are inappropriate. Movement of larger numbers of Medicare recipients into managed care could, almost certainly, reduce government expenditures, and should be encouraged. Additionally, a sound case can be made that—given declining payment rates among private payers—government, as a presumably cost-conscious payer, can and should reduce payment rates accordingly. And finally, a case can certainly be made for requiring a larger financial contribution at least from the higher-income Medicare recipients.

But the point here is that substantial reductions in Medicare/Medicaid expenditures, however desirable or possible, compound and complicate government responsibilities for coverage of the uninsured and for maintenance of a viable safety net. Such cuts reduce the amount of both direct and indirect subsidies to that safety net and the providers who serve it.

Policy Options: The Uninsured, the Safety Net, Medicaid, and Medicare

For advocates of universal coverage (the author included), recommendations for addressing issues of the uninsured, the safety net, and public programs are a depressing undertaking. Universal coverage in some form remains the appropriate response, and its absence a continuing embarrassment in a modern industrialized society.

Short of universal coverage, most approaches to these issues are stopgap measures at best. This section lists a few that deserve exploration.

For the Uninsured

Even if unwilling to impose the requirements necessary to achieve universal coverage, state or federal governments must consider other measures that might ease access to insurance markets for those who might otherwise be uninsured.

1. *Pooling risk:* States (or the federal government) could make sure that individuals had access to small-group pools. If necessary—for political or actuarial reasons—the individual pool could be rated separately from the small-group pool, so that the former did not bear the brunt of the higher-cost individual pool. Additionally, states could consider invoking new opportunities vis a vis ERISA to force larger employers or self-insured employers to pay their share of the higher costs of enrolling individuals in small-group pools.

2. *The New Jersey plan:* As an alternative means of facilitating entry of individuals into insurance markets, state policy makers might review New Jersey's efforts. New Jersey law requires that insurers either participate in the individual market on a community rated, guarantee issue basis, or pay into a risk pool to cover losses of other insurers that do participate. The result has been widespread participation by insurers, and an apparently dramatic increase in the numbers of individuals—many of them previously uninsured—purchasing individual insurance.

3. *Mandated offers:* States could require employers to offer employees access to small-group insurance pools where they exist. The employer need not be required to contribute anything, but the employee would get the advantage of access to the pool—perhaps at group rates. Such an approach might lower the cost of insurance for employed individuals whose employers do not offer insurance, and may entail less of an adverse selection problem than that associated with unemployed individuals.

4. *Unemployment health insurance:* A more radical option would entail adding health insurance to unemployment insurance. A modest increase of perhaps 0.5 percent to 0.75 percent in unemployment insurance costs would enable those who lose jobs and insurance and who are eligible for unemployment benefits to keep their insurance for at least a period of time. While tax increases are never popular, this one would at least be clearly targeted and offer equal protection to all.

5.   *Insurance reform:* The federal government could enact a minimum standard reform law providing protections, including portability for individuals of insurace coverage.

For Medicaid and Medicare

Policy makers also need to explore how changes in the Medicaid and Medicare programs might ease the problem of the uninsured or those who care for them.

1.   *Transition to Medicaid managed care:* Policy makers must be wary of too fast a transition to Medicaid managed care. It is highly unlikely that managed care can save the amounts currently being contemplated. It is also apparent that significant cuts could jeopardize quality.

2.   *Mandatory eligibility increases:* Reductions in Medicaid costs could be used to expand eligibility. Clearly, this runs against 1995 congressional intent; it might even reduce (relative to keeping the savings for other state purposes) the incentives for states to reduce Medicaid expenditures. The incentive problem could probably be addressed with appropriate federal rules; the congressional intent issue is another story.

3.   *Medicaid funds and safety net providers:* State Medicaid programs (or federally imposed rules) could direct some Medicaid recipients to MCOs operated by public or safety net providers, securing these providers some revenue flows, at least for a period of time. Alternatively, states could offer tax incentives, perhaps through definitions of providing community benefit, to MCOs contracting with public providers. Securing private revenues for those providers might, in some circumstances, reduce public costs.

4.   *Cost-cutting via Medicare financial practices:* Medicare might lower costs with more aggressive purchasing strategies. Additionally, moving toward price competition in the Medicare program could reduce government expenditures. Those funds could, congressional policies allowing, be used for a number of safety-net-related purposes. (See discussion in Chapter Eight.)

5.   *A new approach to long-term care:* For a variety of reasons, including rising Medicaid expenditures, policy makers will eventually need to address this issue. One option worth consideration might be a mandated, IRA-type long-term account. All individuals

might be required to put a small percentage of income or wages into a personal or family account to pay long-term care costs. If such care were required, the existence of such funds would reduce Medicaid long-term care costs. If not required for care, the fund would revert to the individual's estate.

Obviously, while requiring a government-imposed mandate, such a proposal would not require individuals to do more than save for their own needs, while having the added benefit of making others do so as well.

For the Safety Net

Finally, policy makers might consider a number of options aimed at strengthening the safety net.

1.   *Medicaid funds:* As discussed in the previous subsection, directing Medicaid funds to public providers and providing incentives for private MCOs to contract with safety net providers would reduce stress on the safety net.

2.   *Nonprofit status requirements:* States or the federal government could tighten rules applying to tax-exempt MCOs and hospitals, requiring clearer demonstrations of provision of community benefit in exchange for tax-exempt status. Rules relating to conversion could also be reviewed to determine if public assets were adequately protected. (See discussion at end of this chapter.) Additional revenues generated could be directed toward safety net services and providers.

3.   *Mandate to serve:* States or the federal government might consider requiring at least some private facilities (inpatient and outpatient) to treat the uninsured. Government might pay costs for those services (presumably at less than private rates, but at least at marginal cost). Such a practice would reduce the need for public facilities and enable a reduction in those facilities, perhaps producing net government savings.

Academic Medical Centers: A Special Case

Like the public safety net, academic medical centers serve important public interests. These include training of health care professionals, leadership in biomedical research, development and provision of breakthrough and high-tech clinical care, and in many cases, participation in the safety net by providing service to uninsured, underinsured, and other vulnerable populations, including Medicaid recipients.

And like many safety net facilities, many academic medical centers are confronting serious challenges that at least in some circumstances may undermine their capacity to perform those public services. Although different in their specifics, many of these challenges stem from developments similar to the challenges faced by safety net facilities outlined earlier—declines in direct and indirect public funding and unique circumstances reducing ability to compete in the new marketplace.

The Challenge to Academic Medical Centers

Academic medical centers, for one thing, may face significant reductions in the funds directed to them through the Medicare program for graduate medical education. By one estimate (probably high) these reductions could total $27 billion over seven years (Blumenthal, 1995). State Medicaid funds that flow to academic medical centers—for educational purposes and for disproportionate amounts of care delivered to underserved populations—are also likely to be reduced, and in some cases have already been reduced.

Overall reductions in Medicaid and Medicare spending will also hit many academic medical centers hard. Proportionately, at least, the Medicaid reductions may be more significant, as many academic medical centers, relative to other hospitals, are disproportionately dependent on Medicaid reimbursements. Institutions wishing to maintain commitments to serve the uninsured will find overall reductions in funds from the public programs particularly painful.

The rise of managed care and the changing marketplace, however, may pose even greater challenges. As states and the federal government seek to invoke managed care as an answer to rising Medicaid and Medicare costs, academic medical centers may find that those populations still free to seek their services may now be compelled to patronize hospitals contracting with their managed care plan. But, for the academic medical center, attaining such contracts may be difficult. Because they tend to attract higher-cost cases, because of the costs associated with education, and for a number of other reasons, average costs per patient (adjusted for case mix) may be 15 percent to 35 percent higher than average in academic medical centers (Blumenthal, 1995). In a fee-for-service marketplace, when patients could enter the hospital of their choice and price competition was less intense, such higher charges might not damage competitive positioning. In that pre-managed-care universe, some of those higher medical costs could be shifted to private payers. But as managed care penetration rises and price competition increases, no amount of reputation can overcome significantly higher costs. The ability to cost-shift declines, and with it the competitive position of the academic medical center. Today, it is generally presumed that a reputation for high-tech expertise and quality in general can command a modest 5 percent to 10 percent addition to competitive prices. But few suggest that reputation can push prices much higher and still retain a competitive posture.

Under some circumstances, even the assets of an academic medical center can become liabilities. An outstanding reputation for cardiac surgery might, under most circumstances, be desirable; but many MCOs may fear that contracting with a hospital bearing such a reputation will attract those (the highest-risk cases) most likely to need those high-cost services.

To these marketplace liabilities can be added a number of factors that, in the view of many, have kept academic medical centers from successfully adjusting to new market realities. Many have been slow to adjust to the paradigm of hospitals as cost centers rather than revenue centers. Some have been reluctant to downsize, to acknowledge that they too must cut costs, or to accept that MCOs are no longer willing to support the higher costs of high-tech, procedure-oriented and specialty-dominated institutions.

The Response of Academic Medical Centers

As a result of these combinations of forces, many academic medical centers face real crises, the outcomes of which are unclear and likely to be determined on a case-by-case basis. But what is clear is that many academic medical centers are employing what assets they have in a wide variety of strategies to assure themselves a successful place in the new marketplace.

In this regard, it is important to emphasize that these institutions maintain high levels of prestige, administrative expertise, and reputations for quality of care, especially in the most critical cases. They have a unique capacity to deliver some of the most complicated and costly of services—often at lower costs due to higher volume—and, perhaps because they have not been pressed to compete, a substantial capacity to reduce costs from current levels. Additionally, despite current public funding reductions and marketplace disadvantages, many remain in very strong financial positions, with large amounts of capital available to invoke networking and other strategies. Those strategies run the gamut from modest adjustment to major overhaul and from short-term cost reduction efforts to the seeking of leadership in the organized systems of the future. In these respects, the strategies being invoked—while generally focused on unique aspects of academic medicine—are not dramatically different from strategies being invoked by other hospitals and health care organizations. In very broad terms these include efforts to improve access to the managed care revenue stream and, in many cases, to position the institutions to perform critical roles in ODSs.

Most obvious of all, many academic medical centers are expanding efforts to improve efficiency and cut costs, including reductions in overall size and in numbers of beds. The University of California Medical Center in San Francisco put plans for a new $39 million cancer treatment center on hold and planned reductions of 550 jobs over an eighteen-month period; the medical center at Duke University planned to combine seventy-nine specialty labs into four general units; the University of Cincinnati adopted standard medical treatment protocols and focused on eliminating unnecessary procedures; the Cleveland Clinic reported reducing operating room costs by 15 percent in 1994 ("Can Academic Health Centers Survive?", 1995). The newly merged Massachusetts General Hospital and Brigham and Women's Hospital plan to eliminate 700 of their more than 1,700 beds over the next five years (Blumenthal, 1995). The numbers of examples are almost limitless.

Academic medical centers have also been aggressive in seeking to expand revenues through the promotion of outpatient services or via product differentiation—emphasizing high-tech services like organ transplants or implementing new clinical programs in women's health and sports medicine.

And most significantly, academic medical centers are spearheading the organization of networks—of hospital systems, of primary care physicians, and of feeder hospitals—and expanding vertical relationships by employing primary care physicians and purchasing primary care practices or entering long-term contracts with MCOs. They are also attempting to strengthen their image as indispensable purveyors of high-quality, high-tech medicine that no MCO should be without, advertising themselves with slogans like "Don't join any HMO unless they have a contract with. . . ." In addition, they are forming their own MCOs and even entering joint ventures with—or allowing themselves to be acquired by—for-profit hospital chains.

Examples of such activities abound. Leaders of the merging Massachusetts General Hospital and Brigham and Women's Hospital expect to establish a vertically integrated ODS including over seven hundred primary care physicians. The University Medical Center at the University of Nevada has decided to form its own HMO. The University of Pennsylvania is investing heavily in the purchase of physician practices. The University of California, Los Angeles, acquired Santa Monica Hospital to strengthen its primary care base and feeder system. Tulane University sold 80 percent of its medical center to Columbia/HCA; Emory University (which rejected an offer from Columbia/HCA) is organizing a statewide network of nearly forty hospitals and up to five thousand physicians that will have a presence in every Georgia market ("Can Academic Health Centers Survive?", 1995). And a number of academic medical centers are participating in a new national network of cancer hospitals with expectations of improving quality and cost-effectiveness of cancer treatment.

There is no way of knowing, at present, which or how many of such efforts will prove successful. Some will most likely result in major organizational leadership roles for academic centers. Others will fail to overcome the obstacles facing these centers, leading to radical changes in function or size, or even to closure.

Whether that success or failure has a larger impact on the public interest may rest on whether or not, in any given circumstance, the outcomes of market change and academic medical center efforts to survive and prosper lead to unacceptable declines in the production of those public services that academic medical centers are uniquely qualified to supply. If, for example, in order to compete, an academic center must substantially scale back its readiness to offer high-quality care to the most vulnerable of populations, then a particular hospital's adjustment may become a community concern. If the need to reduce costs to MCOs results in sizable reductions of research capacity, that, too, may entail substantial public interest costs.

Workforce Considerations

There is also the issue of professional training. Here the public interest may lie less in protecting the services provided by academic medical centers and more in changing those services. Training in academic medical centers has traditionally focused on research and on specialty and inpatient services, whereas the clearly growing needs are for increased training in primary care and management of care in ambulatory care settings.

And there is clearly a substantial difference between training in inpatient and ambulatory settings. The former is more focused on intensive treatment of the sickest patients, often in high-cost, high-tech environments. The latter is more focused on primary care, prevention, and use of the most appropriate provider. It is thus often the more appropriate forum in which to learn principles of cost containment, coordination of care, and population-based health care.

There is, as one analyst labeled it, no "gold standard" for determining the optimal mix of specialty and primary care physicians (Epstein, 1995b). But numerous commissions and studies, as well as unlimited numbers of anecdotal reports, have emphasized the oversupply of specialists, and—in many areas—the undersupply of primary care physicians. There is among policy analysts, at least, consensus that the current mix of about 70 percent specialty, 30 percent primary care is far out of balance (Epstein, 1995b). And the most widely cited study in this regard suggests that in the year 2000 the nation may have about the right number of primary care physicians, but an excess of 150,000 specialists (Epstein, 1995b).

Today there is some evidence that medical schools and residency programs are giving more emphasis to primary care and managed care-related subjects and to training in outpatient and managed care environments. Increasing numbers of medical schools are offering courses on cost and cost containment (not just covering these issues in other courses), and many are expanding training programs in outpatient settings, often as early as the first year in medical school. Yale University, for example, like many others, has made a primary care clerkship a requirement. And whereas no medical school received foundation money to expand primary care courses in 1990, by 1995, fifty schools were in receipt of such grants (Fein, 1995).

There is also some evidence that market realties are affecting the career choices of medical school graduates. In 1992, just 14.6 percent of medical school seniors indicated preferences for careers in primary care, the lowest percentage in history. But in 1995, that figure had almost doubled, to 27.6 percent (Fein, 1995). Finally, although these remain a very small portion of overall medical education funding, a number of states have implemented programs that offer funding support for primary care training.

But, given the realities of how training is financed and to whom the money goes, it seems unlikely that market forces will be sufficient to curtail the growth in the numbers of specialists or sufficiently direct training to ambulatory settings and primary care. The great bulk of training funds come from the Medicare program and go to academic medical centers. Over $6 billion a year in support of direct and indirect medical education costs remains a critical source of funding for these institutions, supporting research activities and constituting a substantial portion of the difference in costs between teaching and nonteaching hospitals (Epstein, 1995b). As a result, these institutions are not likely to readily reduce their numbers of trainees. Nor are they likely to encourage significant changes in specialty/primary care ratios because, for a variety of reasons, specialty training generates greater revenues than training in primary care.

Nor, finally, are they likely to send large numbers of residents outside the hospital for training elsewhere, especially if such an exodus carries with it the approximately $71,000 per trainee that hospitals receive each year for the training. Reports that training in ambulatory settings is more costly and more likely to lead to a loss of productivity only compound the problem.

In sum, even if market lessons compel students into dramatically different choices, significantly reducing the pool of potential trainees in specialty practice, public interest in increased ambulatory training—including practical training in the management and coordination of care—will not be well-served by current training practices and financial arrangements. Somehow, policy makers may need to discover a better compromise between the needs of academic medical centers (which serve both private and public interests) and the public need for an appropriately trained workforce.

The Clinton administration made a substantial effort in this regard as part of its Health Security Act. But its proposal to adjust the numbers and types of residencies clearly reached beyond acceptable levels of regulatory intervention. Today, proposals to impose allocation or regulation formulas would appear to have even less chance of success. Among other things, such proposals would have severe impact on some regions—New York and Massachusetts, most particularly, where medical training is concentrated.

The Health Security Act also included proposals to create an all-payer funding mechanism for graduate medical education, which would have replaced Medicare funding with funds collected from all payers (including MCOs and self-insured employers). This concept still wins support among many policy analysts. But even though the plan would enable government to reduce its costs—shifting them to the private sector—few expect that such a proposal could overcome the obvious political barriers.

What policy makers may be left with, then, is greater targeting of Medicare funds, including increases in funds allotted for primary care training and reductions in payments for training in specialties considered to be in oversupply. Such an approach could stop far short of government allocation of training slots; it would not mandate that academic medical centers change their practices. Rather, it would assert the right of a funder—in this case government with public tax dollars—to pay for what it needed.

Related to this option, obviously, is a reduction in the number of residencies for which Medicare is willing to pay. However, this policy option may be more complicated than it appears. It may be possible to define goals in terms of numbers of physicians needed, but there remains considerable debate over the true costs of physician training.

Another potential option, one that may win widespread public support, would be to limit the number of residency slots that might go to graduates of foreign medical schools. This might be achieved by limiting the number of funded residency positions to 100 percent or 110 percent of the number of U.S. medical school graduates.

Those concerned about safety net facilities and vulnerable populations, however, might be wary of such alternatives. Graduates of these foreign medical schools have traditionally been more likely and more willing to accept modest-paying positions in areas, especially inner cities, that have high concentrations of vulnerable populations.

The Rise of For-Profit Health Care

As detailed in Chapter Four, there has been a substantial movement among MCOs from nonprofit to for-profit status. And while less than 15 percent of hospitals are for-profit corporations, there is not only little question that for-profits are gaining in influence, but also widespread expectation that they will continue to do so.

The rise of the for-profits has much to do with the changing nature of the marketplace. Above all, mergers, acquisitions, practice purchases, expansions of geographic coverage, new information systems, entry into new markets, and the need to be able to survive temporary financial losses in battles for market share place a premium on access to capital. A variety of statutory rules relating to who can pay what to whom and under what circumstances may also advantage for-profit competitors. And for-profits may have greater flexibility to downsize and adjust to changing market forces—and greater pressures imposed on them to do so.

Whatever the cause of the for-profit movement, its potential impact on public interests may be considerable. The most obvious such impact is the potential for a loss of overall system capacity to provide charitable care to those unable to pay for care they require. A second issue relates to the question of whether or not the public is getting appropriately compensated when previously tax-exempt nonprofit insurers or hospitals convert to for-profit status.

For-Profit and Nonprofit MCOs

By 1994, the rise of the for-profit MCO appeared to be a fact written in stone. The market share of for-profit HMOs had risen from 47 percent in 1988 to 58 percent, with one MCO (Kaiser) holding 25 percent of the nonprofit market share. Seventy percent of HMOs were for-profit. Non-HMO MCOs are almost exclusively for-profit. And perhaps most striking of all, in 1994, the rate of enrollment growth in for-profit HMOs (19 percent) was three times the rate (5.8 percent) of nonprofit HMOs (Group Health Association of America, 1995a).

Concerns about the decline in numbers and influence of the for-profit MCO focus on general reservations about increasing responsiveness to short-term stockholder, as opposed to longer-term local community needs. It is presumed, for example, that for-profit MCOs will exert more pressure on affiliated hospitals to improve profits, and thus, perhaps, to reduce the provision of charity care. Those expressing concerns are also generally quick to cite the rise of commercial insurers and of national rather than local, independent MCOs. As a result, concerns about the rise of for-profit MCOs become part of a larger concern regarding the corporatization of health care, a concept that—while ill-defined—is hardly without significance.

Other analysts, even some who see advantages in conversion to for-profit status, express concerns about the speed of the nonprofit decline, fearing that too little is known about the potential impact of that decline. There may be no significant problem, they assert. But the speed of the change may be such that its negative effects won't be understood until the proverbial water is already under the bridge (Tokarski, 1994).

Finally, many—especially consumer group leaders—express concern that the public may not be receiving appropriate compensation for nonprofit assets.

Overall, however, most analysts express only modest concern about the rise of for-profit MCOs. The general lack of concern tends to reflect an assessment that—with the exception of some group or staff model HMOs—the differences between for-profit and nonprofit MCOs, at least from the consumer or employer point of view, are minimal to nonexistent. Moreover, it is argued that as states move toward insurance reforms and community rating, one of the major distinctions between for-profit and nonprofit plans (community rating by the latter) will be less relevant.

Nor does there appear to be compelling evidence that nonprofit MCOs score higher on consumer satisfaction ratings. For example, with regard to consumer perceptions of quality, a recent survey of federal employees found virtually no difference in quality between for-profit and nonprofit plans. Ninety percent of enrollees in both for and nonprofit plans rated their plan "good, very good, or excellent" on quality (Center for the Study of Services, 1995).[1]

For-profit MCOs, obviously, also generate tax revenues. And while some long-standing group or staff models may provide true community benefit, anecdotal reports suggest that those MCOs more likely to convert have been those less likely to provide such benefits. In such cases, to put it bluntly, the public might as well take the money.

Finally, there are many who view going public not just as the absence of a negative but as clearly positive development. While consumer groups may fear the impact of stockholder pressures to pursue the bottom line, advocates of for-profit status suggest that it is precisely that bottom-line pressure that renders for-profits more efficient and—particularly relevant in today's health care marketplace—more willing to engage in the downsizing necessary throughout the system.

For-Profit and Nonprofit Hospitals: A More Contentious Debate

Relative to concerns regarding the conversion of MCOs, concerns about the apparent reduction of influence in the nonprofit hospital sector are far more intense and widespread.

This is a debate in large part over values, but it is somewhat muddied and complicated by confusion and misconceptions regarding what is actually happening in the hospital sector. On the one hand, while the general perception of changing ownership status is one of rapid and substantial change, the actual decline in the percentage of hospitals that are nonprofit is modest. On the other hand, it is clear that the dramatic growth of Columbia/HCA and

---

[1]This was not a scientific survey, but did receive a 60 percent response rate.

its recent direction toward acquisitions of nonprofits, the greater profits being experienced by for-profit as opposed to nonprofit hospital systems, and the advantages of those with greater access to capital in a time of considerable merger an acquisition activity, all point to growing influence for the for-profit sector.

During the first six months of 1994, reportedly, for- profit companies announced the acquisition of forty-seven nonprofit hospitals (Freudenheim, 1995a)—certainly a sizable number, but still only around 1 percent of the nation's nonprofit community hospitals. It is also reported that dozens of nonprofits have rejected acquisition or joint venture offers from for-profit chains. Overall, most observers assume there will be at least some increase in the numbers of for-profit hospitals and in their influence. But beyond that point consensus collapses, both as to the extent of for-profit growth and influence anticipated, and even more as to the impact of such growth on public purposes and needs. Our focus here is on the latter question.

Those concerned with current trends focus primarily on the capacity of the system to deliver care to the needy, especially at a time when the numbers of the uninsured continue to mount. While most recognize that many nonprofit hospitals function very much like for-profits, it is also widely acknowledged that many provide significant levels of public benefit, especially charity care. This is especially true of many religion-based hospitals, academic medical centers, and publicly owned facilities.

A significant decline in the nonprofit sector, then, might obviously reduce system capacity to deliver charity care. For example, in the most comprehensive review of conversion outcomes, a 1986 Institute of Medicine report found that hospitals that had converted to for-profit status increased profitability by, among other things, reducing Medicaid loads and charity care ("A Delicate Balancing Act," 1995).

And a recent study by *Modern Healthcare* (Burda, 1995) found, in a study of Tennessee hospitals, that private nonprofit hospitals provided about 10 percent more uncompensated care than for-profits. (These figures do not include public hospitals, which provide the greatest amounts of charitable care.)

Interestingly, in terms of delivery of uncompensated care, Columbia's/HCA's hospitals were on the low side, even when compared to other for-profits; seven of the nine Columbia hospitals reviewed were below the mean in terms of delivery of uncompensated care delivered by for-profits.[2]

Reduced levels of charitable care from private nonprofit hospitals would increase pressure on public hospitals and safety nets. These institutions, already under budgetary stress, would have to absorb a greater charity load, reducing their already limited capacity to compete and increasing their current distress.

Even should the numbers of hospitals converting to for-profit status remain minimal, increasing competition on price and for shares of managed care contracts can put pressure on nonprofit hospitals to reduce levels of charity care, the costs of which may less easily be shifted to other payers. Moreover, those nonprofit hospitals that maintain community commitments may find themselves at a competitive disadvantage. Legal restrictions that limit the ability of nonprofits to merge, purchase practices, establish PHOs, or operate POS plans could add to that competitive disadvantage.

Additionally, even if calculations of the trend to for-profit status may be exaggerated at a nationwide level, a regional market analysis often reveals a different reality. In some markets, for-profits own much more than 15 percent of hospitals or beds. For example, Columbia/HCA alone owns 25 percent of hospitals in Florida. In such markets, significant declines in the nonprofit sector could potentially place considerable stress on safety net capacities.

Finally, many express concerns that partnership activities and joint ventures that involve for-profit and nonprofit hospitals may mask the extent of decline in the influence of nonprofits (and of the nonprofit ethic). The nonprofit legal structure may remain. But the driving force behind the enterprise may begin to undergo subtle—and not-so-subtle—transformations.

On the other hand, a solid case can be mounted that the extent of community loss resulting from a decline in the nonprofit hospital sector has been greatly exaggerated. For one

[2]However, the study did not factor in taxes paid by for-profits, some of which could provide state and federal governments with funds to cover the needy. Columbia's Tennessee hospitals report paying $30 million in state taxes, while total uncompensated care in the state (116 hospitals) was $502.8 million.

thing, a distinction might be drawn between charitable nonprofits (most notably religious institutions) and other nonprofits.
Those nonprofits most likely to convert, it can be argued, are
already functioning much like for-profits. Loss of charity care
from such conversions would be minimal, and tax revenues
would increase.

Many argue along this line that the definition of "community
benefits" (an undefined requirement including such things as
acceptance of Medicaid patients, open emergency rooms, and provision of charitable care) that nonprofits must meet to maintain
tax-exempt status is too lax, or not enforced with adequate vigor.
Large numbers of nonprofit hospitals, it is asserted, do not offer
enough community benefit to justify their tax exemption. The
movement to Medicaid managed care may render such justification even more difficult. As more Medicaid enrollees move into
private MCOs, with hospitals being paid negotiated rates, the rationale for offering tax-exempt status to those accepting more Medicaid enrollees will grow more tenuous.

And those tax advantages involve considerable sums. The estimated 1994–1998 cost to the federal government of allowing tax
deductible contributions to nonprofit hospitals is $8.8 billion. The
cost of allowing them to issue tax-exempt bonds is an additional
$10.8 billion (Boisture, 1994). And these totals do not include
losses associated with federal income tax exemptions or local property tax exemptions.[3] Viewed from another perspective, the tax
advantages of the nonprofits may amount to between 5 percent
and 8 percent of revenues (Boisture, 1994; Bradford Gray, interview, 1995). In no state, according to one authority, do the differences between for-profits and nonprofits on uncompensated care
amount to that much money. Thus, dollars gained via taxes could
pay for services lost in reductions of uncompensated care (Bradford Gray, interview, 1995). (Of course, those concerned about

---

[3]There are no official estimates on the revenue loss associated with the federal
income tax or local property tax exemptions. Some believe that losses from the
former would be modest, and that most nonprofits are break-even operations.
Others note the large reserves of some nonprofits and draw different conclusions.
Losses to local property tax revenues are probably substantial, given the capital-
intensive nature of hospital operations (Boisture, 1994).

losses in charitable care will derive little comfort from exchanges of that care for tax revenues—unless, that is, the revenues are used to replace the lost care.)

Given these realities, a number of states—including Massachusetts, Pennsylvania, and Texas—have recently undertaken efforts to assess the amount of charitable care being provided by nonprofits and to require them to pay their share of local and state taxes. A new Texas law, for example, imposes a charity care assessment equal to 4 percent of net patient revenue on nonprofit hospitals (Tokarski, 1994).

Moreover, conversion need not lead to a total loss in delivery of charitable care. Foundations established with the conversion of public to private assets can provide community service, including funds to replace charity care once delivered by the nonprofit hospital. Conversions can even involve guarantees for the provision of ongoing charitable care. For example, in its 1985 acquisition of Wesley Medical Center in Wichita, Kansas, the Hospital Corporation of America agreed to maintain levels of charity care ("A Delicate Balancing Act," 1995). Such guarantees could also be mandated by government.

Finally, there may be good reason to question the public policy of providing tax-exempt status to hospitals—including tax advantages for capital construction—when there is already a widely acknowledged excess in hospital capacity. Many would prefer to see tax breaks or government expenditures targeted more directly at the delivery of charitable care, or at the creation of outpatient and community facilities where needed.

Conversions and Community Assets

When nonprofit MCOs or hospitals convert to for-profit status, federal and state laws generally dictate that the organization donate to charity the value of its assets, which—as a result of favored tax status—are considered to be owned by the community. Such conversions, whether occurring through mergers, acquisitions, or spinoffs from parent organizations, are raising significant issues regarding the valuation of community assets, and the use and control of those assets by the foundations and trusts established as a result of the conversion process.

For a number of reasons, these issues are likely to begin appearing with increasing frequency on political and legislative radar screens. If nothing else, conversions can be enormously complex transactions, involving state and federal statutes on fraud and abuse, tax-exempt status, conversion law, inurement, Stark laws and others.

Far more important than the complexity are the amounts of money involved—or, to put it more accurately, the amounts of money that might, but haven't always been, involved. In a number of perhaps many cases, it appears, those once-public assets may have been significantly undervalued, with health organizations converting to for-profit enterprises that soon had stock value of vastly greater amounts than conversion evaluation figures had suggested (Bailey, 1994; Rundle, 1995a). See Table 10.1 for some examples of health organizations that may have given less to charity than their full value.

As a result, state regulators—who often maintain considerable discretion in how they evaluate public assets—have been increasingly pressed by consumer groups and others to take more aggressive postures in the evaluation process. In a number of more recent conversions, regulators have veered away from past practices, in which they tended to rely on consultants who supplied figures that often turned out to be far below actual market value (Rundle, 1995a).

In the words of California's Commissioner of Corporations, Gary S. Mendoza, states need stricter rules to "make sure that the nonprofit health groups give 100 percent of their assets to charity when they become for-profit, and that charities benefit from future increases in the value of the new non-profit" (Bailey, 1994). In one particularly precedent-setting decision, Mendoza argued that Blue Cross should use the market value of its 80 percent stockholding in Wellpoint as the basis for its charitable contribution. In March 1996, after several years of negotiation with regulators, California Blue Cross agreed to provide about $3 billion in cash and stock to two new foundations (Freudenheim, 1996). If followed in other states, this practice could lead to dramatic increases in the evaluation of assets, and thus in the amount of funds to be donated to charity. Consumer groups prefer approaches like this one, including the prospect of tying the future value of foundation holdings to the stock price of the new for-profit. In this way, should the value of the assets have been underestimated, the foundation and public holdings it represents are not short-changed. As an additional means of

Table 10.1. Is Something Getting Lost?

Converting Organization	Conversion Date	Charity Donation at Time of Conversion or Sale (dollars)	Later Value or Sale Price (dollars)	Value 1993–1994 (dollars)
PacifiCare Health Systems	1984	360,000	45.3 million (1985)	2.2 billion
FHP International	1984	38.5 million	135.6 million	1.87 billion
Group/Health Plan of Greater St. Louis	1985	4 million	40 million	46.2 million
Foundation Health Plan	1984	78 million	302.4 million (1991)	1.9 billion
Presbyterian/St. Lukes Healthcare Corp., Denver	1985	123 million	180 million	NA
Inland Health Care Loma Linda, Ca.	1985	663,000	37.5 million (1986)	NA
Health Net Woodland Hills, Ca.	1992	300 million	300 million	1.7 billion

Adapted from Bailey, 1994; Rundle, 1995a.

preventing underevaluations, especially in the case where current managers and purchasers are one and the same, consumer groups argue that the converting organizations should be put up for bid, a more market-sensitive mechanism of determining their actual value.

And, most important, there is a noticeable increase in conversion activity that may involve very large sums. This is especially true in the managed care sector, where conversion activity has been more dramatic and converting organizations of considerable greater value. Over the past ten years, dozens of foundations have been created as the result of conversions of MCOs or hospitals, many involving amounts in the hundreds of millions, and a few—resulting from recent California MCO conversions ranging into the $1–$2 billion (and now $3 billion) range, creating some of the nation's largest philanthropies. Moreover, the potential conversion of a number of the nation's sixty-eight Blue Cross and Blue Shield plans (with almost sixty-five million enrollees and reported assets of approximately $32 billion) has obvious potential to raise the visibility of conversion-related issues. It is hardly shocking then, that, as noted in Chapter Four, conversions of MCOs over the next ten years could involve "tens of billions" (Rundle, 1995b).

For all these reasons, the recent growth in health organization conversion activity has led to a host of policy questions. How, for one thing, should assets of converting organizations be evaluated? As noted, different approaches can produce huge differences in funds to be delivered to foundations. Another series of issues surrounds the question of control over and independence of the new foundations. When a hospital conversion leaves a new foundation with part-ownership in the now for-profit hospital, for example, conflicts can arise when board members sit on the board of the foundation and of the hospital. Charges have arisen in such contexts to the effect that foundation leaders, in expending foundation resources, were favoring their hospital partner or refusing to issue grants to competing nonprofit hospitals.

Still another series of questions focuses on the best use of foundation funds. Foundations established via conversions of hospitals, it is asserted (especially those with a stake in the hospital), may be prone to keep charitable dollars in service to the hospital, perhaps for the provision of charitable care. Especially if the foundation is linked to the hospital, its board may have less interest in shifting trust dollars to nonhospital (community clinic and out-patient) services. While such a shift in focus might, in some cases, more directly address community needs, it might also lead to hospital downsizing or even closure.

For-Profit Status Conversions and Public Policy

Given the amounts and health care stakes involved, such issues are receiving unacceptably low levels of attention from policy makers. At minimum, these issues—from the impact of a potential decline in the nonprofit hospital sector, to the trade-offs between community service and government revenue losses, to the issues of public assets in conversion processes—require considerably greater public airing. And, as was suggested in the case of antitrust policy, that airing must occur among policy makers, not regulators or judges. These are issues of value, in which benefits and risks of potential decisions need to be weighed against each other in the broadest possible context. That is the stuff of public policy, not regulation.

In particular, states and the federal government need to review the issue of community benefits and whether or not—given the revenue losses involved—MCOs or hospitals are providing service justifying their tax advantages. Means by which those truly providing a public benefit can be distinguished from those providing no such benefit need to be evaluated and applied—with appropriate rewards and appropriate losses of privilege distributed accordingly.

More aggressive efforts to monitor conflicts of interest between for-profit hospitals and MCOs and the foundations they have established may also be of value. So too may be consideration of means by which nonprofit organizations or foundations are encouraged to direct more funds toward safety net, outpatient, and community needs as opposed to inpatient needs. Included in such a review, of course, should be the question of the extent to which current tax policy is encouraging the flow of public assets toward less than the most pressing public needs.

Such policies might result either in more funds being directed at areas of greater public need, or in greater government revenues—which could, in turn, be directed at the most critical needs. Here, however, may lie a problem. If revenues raised by tightening community benefit standards aren't utilized to support charitable care and other community needs (for example, if they are used for deficit reduction), community benefit programs could suffer a net loss.

The surge in conversion activity, its expected continuing expansion, and the amounts involved in such transactions, also demand heightened public scrutiny. As discussed, the issue is not just one of accurately assessing the value of public assets; it is also one of determining how those assets should be used and who should make those determinations. With the system's capacity to deliver charitable care being threatened, with the focus of care shifting from inpatient to outpatient facilities, with the numbers of the uninsured continuing to rise, and with government likely to reduce its support of safety-net-related spending, the need to make optimal use of public resources seems ever more important.

In sum, it is very possible that, via tax advantages and less-than-aggressive monitoring of conversion processes, there is a great deal of essentially public money involved here, the spending of which may not be serving the greatest public needs. Governments need to find out how much is involved, and the extent to which such an accusation may be accurate.

Finally, government may wish to review a variety of statutes that—often with appropriate economic rationale—may render it more difficult for nonprofit organizations to compete in the changing marketplace. If such statutes—for example fraud and abuse laws and rules on private inurement—are generating a movement on the part of nonprofit organizations to for-profit status, and if this movement is deemed undesirable, some means may be required to moderate the impact of these statutes.

Conclusion

In the marketplace of public opinion, managed care, and prepaid health care in particular, start out behind the proverbial eight ball. To most consumers, the concept that organizations and providers can make more by doing less establishes an inherent conflict of interest between patient and system needs. Inevitably, many believe, incentives to do less will be something other than incentives to improve efficiency and cost-effectiveness; they will be incentives to do less than what should be done.

The conflict is real, but the level of concern stems in large part from misunderstandings regarding the operation and failings of the now-fading fee-for-service alternative.

Most significantly, that alternative was marked by significant overutilization of services. Eventually, researchers began to identify and understand this overutilization and the higher costs and threats to quality it entailed. Indeed, today there is far more proof of fee-for-service doing too much than there is of managed care doing too little.

But most consumers saw neither the cost nor shortcomings of quality in the old system. Soaring premiums were paid (or at least were perceived to be paid) by employers; bills were paid by insurers. As for quality, it was difficult (and still is) for the public to view doing too much as an issue of quality. And given that they didn't see the costs of fee-for-service and didn't perceive overutilization (if they saw it at all) as a problem, the finding that managed care can produce the same or better quality with much lower utilization was of relatively little value or meaning to most consumers. What they saw first, and continue to see in managed care, are restrictions, denials, and reduced choice. If managed care had something to sell then, it was to employers, not consumers.

Additionally, in critically evaluating the incentive of MCOs to do less, many consumers seemed to forget that traditional insurers had and have the same incentives in offering fee-for-service plans; they are just less apparent. In fee-for-service medicine, to be sure, physicians may have no direct incentive to do less, and appearances of physician-patient conflict of interest are, therefore, less than in managed care arrangements. But on the insurer side, fee-for-service insurers, just like HMOs, make more when they pay out less. In this regard, many consumers may be quick to forget the claims that were denied because "the procedure wasn't deemed necessary," or was considered "experimental," or wasn't "authorized." They may also forget the many claims that were paid only in part, because the physician charged more than the "usual and customary" fee—for which, of course, there was no usual and customary definition. Finally, consumers may forget, or may not have realized, that as more fee-for-service systems adopted more managed care cost containment strategies, these kinds of rejections and denials were growing more commonplace.

The combination of the obvious do-less/make-more conflict inherent in the managed care construct and the failure to see flaws in the fee-for-service construct have left managed care with an almost herculean public relations problem. As one expert in consumer protection described it, when a patient receives poor care from a physician in the fee-for-service system, they blame the physician, not the system (that is, the insurance system or payment system, for example) in which the physician functions. But when a patient receives poor care from a physician in an HMO, they are more likely to blame the HMO and even the whole concept of managed care. Thus, every anecdote is a potential example (perhaps even a news story) of systemic failure.

In short, managed care and HMOs in particular have gotten a bit of a bum rap. They may not have achieved their full potential, and they may entail inherent conflicts of interest the outcomes of which need to be monitored. But they should not be compared to an idealized system that wasn't what people thought it was, that proved itself almost wholly incapable—at least in the absence of regulated fees—of controlling costs, and that did not offer—especially when doing more than necessary is viewed as a negative—better quality of care.

This may be especially true when we consider the potential of the emerging MCO, which is—unlike many of the earlier managed care networks—more likely to include a larger element of organization. The new partnerships emerging and the greater capacity of those partnerships to accept financial and clinical accountability for patient care have the potential to both lower price and improve quality of care. Specifically, as the foregoing analysis has tried to suggest, the mature MCO—whether invoking ownership or contractual relationships—has a greater potential to achieve economies of scale and administrative savings; improve coordination of care over the full range of medical services including services for the chronically ill; expand and make greater use of administrative and clinical information services; achieve the proper balance (perhaps a moving target) between primary care and specialty services; develop innovative approaches to organizational structure and coordination of care; increase incentives for improvement of preventive care and overall health status of the enrolled population; generate and collect data on performance and outcomes against which they be evaluated; make better use of nonphysician providers and lower cost and outpatient settings, including home health care services; and improve performance—through use of guidelines, improved physician selection procedures, and ongoing education efforts—of providers and of the system as a whole.

But the existence of capacity and potential for positive change are no guarantee that the potential will be achieved. Today, that potential—especially with regard to clinical integration and quality of care—remains largely untapped. And there is no certainty that it will be fully tapped.

The questions to be asked, then, are (1) What factors will be most critical in determining whether or not the potential will be achieved? (2) Recalling that there is no such thing as "no government health care policy," how might public policy support—by intervention or nonintervention—the achievement of that potential?

By way of summary, four critical areas stand out.

Maintaining a Competitive Environment

Ascertaining the ideal level of government intervention in market mechanisms is a persistent challenge in free-market economies. Government intervention may be required to establish rules of the game (for example, limit the rights of insurers to drop enrollees), to impose minimal requirements on competitors (for example, solvency and licensure standards), level the competitive playing field (for example, reduce allowable levels of experience rating), and to accomplish other objectives. Most important of all—especially in an age of consolidation—government intervention may be required, via antitrust enforcement and other means to maintain competition.

Acknowledging the complexity of the regulatory balancing act makes it no easier. Every step of government intervention is likely to be controversial and to attract legitimate concern as well as a healthy dose of hostile rhetoric.

In today's health care marketplace the toughest questions may center around the rate and extent of consolidation activity. As advocated earlier, antitrust enforcement agencies are probably correct in deeming most consolidation and joint venture efforts to be procompetitive. But the potential pace and impact of these efforts suggests the need for improved analytical tools and for broader public discussion regarding potential trade-offs between the values and dangers of consolidation activity under different circumstances and in different sectors.

From a competition point of view, the kinds of vertical integration that are occurring are less of a threat. Arrangements here are less likely to involve competitors. Yet, if many flowers are to bloom, policy makers need to revisit statutes or regulations that may inhibit that flowering. If innovation and coordination are to be encouraged—or at least allowed room to experiment—rules that unnecessarily (admittedly a loaded term) restrict who may employ whom, or own what, or refer to whom, or perform what service under what circumstances need to be reviewed. Some may be absolutely appropriate. Others may seem less relevant in age of managed care and more geared to protect consumers in a fee-for-service marketplace. Rules involving consolidation and integration activities among nonprofits may also benefit from review and/or adjustment, especially if found to reduce the competitive prospects of these organizations.

The fostering of a competitive marketplace may also suggest that policy makers resist the pleas of those who would impose restrictions or limitations on competitive offerings. While often drawing widespread public and media support, laws that demand that MCOs offer "freedom of choice," or point-of-service options, or that they abide by any-willing-provider rules may restrict the types of offerings in the marketplace—offerings, it should be noted, that would not long survive if they cannot attract reasonable levels of purchaser interest.

Policy makers must also wrestle with the insurance regulation question of who can offer what product. The appeal of direct contracting or of provider service networks servicing Medicare beneficiaries may be considerable. Such approaches can enhance competition and maximize consumers' ability to select providers from among known, local competitors. But, clearly, solvency issues arise here, as do issues of an unlevel playing field, in which provider networks get to escape the rules imposed on insurers. Finding the balance here will be difficult, but it may be worth looking for.

Finally, maintaining a competitive environment in an insurance marketplace means that government must address the issues of risk-selection and market segmentation. Unless expressly prohibited from doing so, most insurers will inevitably be drawn into a competition on risk-selection in which there is little public value. This will be especially true as more Medicare and Medicaid recipients move into managed care plans.

Thus, maintaining a competitive insurance marketplace means the imposition of rules that restrict or eliminate competition on risk-selection and that, as a result, foster competition on price and quality The more competition moves in this direction, the more likely it is that systems truly improving performance in health care delivery will be advantaged and rewarded.

Quality and Consumer Protection

The issue here concerns both the ceiling and the floor. The rise of managed care and of the ODS can, in the best of worlds, raise the ceiling—enhancing quality through improved coordination of care, greater attention to prevention and a variety of other means. On the other hand, in the worst of scenarios, capitation and other risk-sharing incentives, can heighten risks of undertreatment, especially for the most vulnerable of patients.

And while it appears likely that today's marketplace will inspire ongoing competition on price, relying on competition to improve quality remains a dicier proposition. As discussed in Chapter Eight, all too often quality remains a matter of perception and a stepchild to the more tangible realities of price. Moreover, the employers in charge of purchasing decisions may consider quality only up to a point, beyond which price clearly rules.

With regard to the ceiling, the inability to compare systems on quality reduces the incentives on those systems to raise quality goals and standards, and to maximize their potential to achieve those goals and standards. Enhanced capacity to evaluate system performance and to compare competing systems would, as outlined earlier, be of great value in encouraging quality improvement. So, too, might be greater emphasis on individual—as opposed to employer— choice of insurance plan, especially if the ultimate choice were between locally identifiable delivery systems as opposed to nationally known coordinators of provider networks.

With regard to the quality floor, one can certainly envision how managed care arrangements and ODSs can enhance quality for the sickest of enrollees—by improving the coordination of care over a continuum of services and among a series of providers, and by promoting prevention and monitoring strategies aimed at reducing the need for hospitalization and other high cost interventions. On the other hand, the potential for underservice—especially of the mentally ill, or of very low-income enrollees—cannot be denied, and there is documentation that, at least in some cases, the drive to lower system costs can threaten the responsibility to provide quality care. The need for protection of the floor may also auger for caution in (although not rejection of) the rapid expansion of Medicaid managed care, especially where state regulatory capacities are limited. It may also suggest a need for such policies as enhanced efforts to monitor disenrollment from insurance plans, and more aggressive monitoring (perhaps including mandatory disclosure) of certain kinds of risk-sharing arrangements.

Purchasing

If consumers are to rely on a competitive marketplace for producing greater value, and especially if there is resistance to aggressive government intervention in that marketplace, the purchaser must be up to the task. As has been argued, the MCO has been, at least in the recent past, something of an ally of the demand side in this regard, bringing pressures on providers to lower costs. Whether or not it will continue to do so in the future is unclear. In markets where exclusive relationships between insurers and providers emerge, or where ODSs emerge as the primary actors, purchasers may be facing a more consolidated—even if more competitive—cast of suppliers. In short, however, although many purchasers may have improved their capacities in the changing marketplace, their organizational efforts pale before those of the provider community. As levels of excess supply decline and as provider organizations grow stronger the supply side may—perhaps via different strategies and arrangements than was the case ten to fifteen years ago—reassert itself.

Thus, the strengthening of the purchaser is likely to remain absolutely critical in the search for value. Insurance reforms that level the competitive playing field appear essential here, lest market segmentation be allowed to reassert itself and pit consumers against each other. Purchasing cooperatives also appear to be an increasingly valuable tool, especially for smaller employers, and government may need to play a role in encouraging their formation or at least in establishing some rules that level the field on which cooperatives play.

Additionally, as managed competition advocates have asserted, the search for value in purchasing should be enhanced as individuals select their insurance plans and are rendered more cost-conscious in that selection process. Enhanced consumer cost-consciousness should result in greater rewards for MCOs that improve value. It should also give consumers—as purchasers and as the ultimate policy makers—a richer awareness of the relationships among price, service, value, and benefits in health care. A public that has a better understanding of these relationships may be more capable of addressing difficult questions of technological advance and trade-offs between benefits and costs.

Beyond the Market

Finally, it must be recognized that a more efficient and more competitive health care marketplace may still leave some out in the proverbial cold. Indeed, as marketplace change and government policy eliminate indirect subsidies while failing to replace them with direct subsidies, the numbers in the cold are likely to grow. Several policies might restrain such growth. These include insurance market reforms that give high-cost, small employer groups access to community rates; extensions of guaranteed issue and community rating rules to individual markets; providing access for individuals to small group or government pools; elimination of pre-existing condition restrictions, at least for those with ongoing insurance coverage; or even the inclusion of health insurance in the unemployment insurance program.

None of these proposals (with the possible exception of the last proposal, a tax) will make a dramatic difference in the numbers of the uninsured. The inability to pay for insurance coverage remains the primary reason individuals cannot access the insurance marketplace. Without substantial subsidies—perhaps combined with mandates—the numbers of the uninsured and of the need for a safety net to provide services to them are not going to decline.

Should policy makers choose to address the subsidy issue (and some, clearly, would prefer not to) at least three broad option areas are available. First, the apparent coming reduction in indirect subsidies could be moderated. Clearly, the largest such subsidies come via the Medicare and Medicaid programs. Substantial cuts in these programs are almost certain to have negative impacts on the numbers of the uninsured and on safety net providers, including academic medical centers. This would prove to be true, it should be emphasized, even if the proposed cuts might have no negative effects on the Medicare and Medicaid programs themselves.

Alternatively, policy makers could find other means of providing safety-net subsidies. For example, states or the federal government could use tax or other policy means to require or offer incentives to insurers or providers to offer higher levels of charitable care. Similar requirements or incentives could be used to encourage insurers or provider systems to contract with public providers. Or, in a means bordering on direct subsidy approaches, all insurers, including self-insuring employers, could be mandated to provide some charitable care or to contribute—via a bed tax or other means—to those who do provide it.

Finally, government could provide more direct subsidies to address the issues of the uninsured or the safety net. Such subsidies could be provided to individuals for the purchase of insurance, to providers who deliver charitable care, or even to employers to encourage them to provide insurance (although this has not generally been found to be very productive unless the subsidies are large and guaranteed over a long term). Obviously, political forces being what they are today, such direct subsidies appear to have the slimmest chance of enactment.

Beyond Insurance to Health Status: The Potential for Public-Private Partnerships

A number of marketplace developments discussed in the foregoing analysis appear to suggest a potential for public-private partnerships. For one thing, as MCOs and delivery systems consolidate into larger units that assume clinical and financial responsibility for the care of larger populations, they may be more prone to extend their focus beyond disease prevention to injury prevention, and to programs aimed at educating enrollees on alcohol and drug abuse, nutrition, or sexually transmitted disease. In short, they may begin to focus greater attention on questions associated with community health status, or public health. Some analysts suggest, in fact, that it is in these realms wherein lies some of the greatest potential for long-term reductions in health costs, all of which may be especially relevant as managed care systems enroll higher numbers of Medicaid recipients.

Especially where consolidation results in a small number of plans or delivery systems—each enrolling large populations—the potential for mutually beneficial public-private sector joint ventures on public health-related issues may be substantial. Jointly sponsored education projects, immunization projects, school-based clinic projects, and alcohol- and drug-related projects might all be candidates for such endeavors.

Another obvious potential area for such cooperation is in data collection. As was discussed in Chapter Eight there may be considerable value in cooperation, especially among purchasers, but also between purchasers and suppliers, on questions of what data needs to be collected, by whom, and for what purposes. Government, as a major purchaser but also as a source of research and financial support for such ventures, seems to be an appropriate facilitator or supporter of such projects. Similar opportunities for joint public-private collaboration abound in the area of health services research—on clinical guidelines and outcomes. As discussed in Chapter Eight, this research is best undertaken with public support because it serves public interests to keep results of such research in the public domain. But such research, whatever the funding source, needs the participation of private delivery systems thus almost mandating a joint public-private effort.

Not only could public and private sectors cooperate on data collection needs, they could also well consider joint purchasing efforts. Suggestions, for example, have been made that the federal employees health benefits program be opened, under some circumstances, to private employers. If concerns exist regarding the financial impacts of merging pools, rates for pools could be separated, while both received the benefits of greater market leverage and reductions in administrative costs. In a similar fashion, local governments and private employers could consider joint purchasing arrangements.

Finally, a number of issue areas discussed would benefit considerably from more extensive public airing in which public and private sectors should participate. These include antitrust, and the ongoing challenge of assessing potential implications of various organizational and market developments for both improved efficiency and competition; the trend toward for-profit ownership of HMOs and hospitals and the means of determining the worth of converting organizations; and the fostering of direct contracting options for providers and purchasers, including the consumer protection measures that may need to accompany such provisions.

Opportunity and Limitation

Those who suggest they know where the health care marketplace is going may be effective at gaining attention. Their bravado may even generate a higher consulting fee.

But, in most cases, they would be getting more attention and fees than they deserve. Even with the increasing amount of analysis being directed at changing marketplaces, it remains difficult to separate trend from best practice, best practice from benchmark, and benchmark from unique circumstance. The tendency of marketplace chatter to exaggerate the rise or breadth of trends only raises the level of confusion.

Which is hardly to suggest that major change is not occurring. (Those who would argue such a conclusion deserve no fees at all.) But it does suggest that many new arrangements, partnerships, and strategies are emerging and are likely to continue emerging in the foreseeable future. Which types of arrangements will come to dominate remains unclear; and when some do, it may be for only a brief period of time.

Such change, of course, will be unsettling for many—especially those whose livelihoods are most directly at stake. But, overall, the changes occurring are overdue, and offer considerable potential to yield positive results in lower costs and higher quality care.

Still, the changes may pose stiff challenges for policy makers, and those challenges will have to be addressed. In doing so, policy makers may well wish to define the overriding goal as maximizing the positive potential of those marketplace changes. And they may wish to define the most appropriate strategy as one of allowing and encouraging, as opposed to directing or regulating, those changes. But even the adoption of a predominantly hands-off approach will not eliminate the need for some new public policies or for the adjustment or elimination of old ones. Much as some might like it to be the case, there is no inevitability to the achievement of harmony between private and public interests.

Appendix

The individuals listed herein provided the author with invaluable information and analysis. The author is indebted to them for their time and for their insight.

Ron Barkley
Publisher, Consultant
Los Angeles, California

Judith Bell
Consumers Union, Inc.
San Francisco, California

Robert E. Bloch
Attorney
Washington, D.C.

Peter Boland
Consultant
Berkeley, California

Lawrence D. Brown
School of Public Health,
   Columbia University
New York, New York

Patricia Butler
Consultant
Boulder, Colorado

Nancy Chockley
National Institute for Health
   Care Management
Washington, D.C.

Gary Claxton
Lewin/VHI
Alexandria, Virginia

William Conway, Jr. M.D.
Henry Ford Health System
Detroit, Michigan

Richard E. Curtis
Institute for Health Policy
   Solutions
Washington, D.C.

Joseph M. Davis
The Medimetrix Group
Cleveland, Ohio

Arnold M. Epstein, M.D.
School of Medicine, Harvard
   University
Cambridge, Massachusetts

Lynn Etheredge
Consultant
Bethesda, Maryland

Barry Fake
Attorney
Fairfax, Virginia

Donald Fisher
American Group Practice
 Association
Alexandria, Virginia

Peter D. Fox
Consultant
Chevy Chase, Maryland

Irene Frazier
Agency for Health Care Policy
 and Research
Rockville, Maryland

Jon Gabel
Group Health Association of
 America
Washington, D.C.

David Gans
Medical Group Management
 Association
Denver, Colorado

Sherry Glied
School of Public Health,
 Columbia University
New York, New York

Bill Gold
Consultant
New York, New York

Marsha R. Gold
Mathematica Policy Research,
 Inc.
Washington, D.C.

Jeff C. Goldsmith
Consultant
Deerfield, Illinois

Peter N. Grant
Attorney
San Francisco, California and
Seattle, Washington

Martin Hickey, M.D.
Lovelace Health System
Albuquerque, New Mexico

Edward Hirschfeld
American Medical
 Association
Chicago, Illinois

Brent James, M.D.
Intermountain HealthCare
Salt Lake City, Utah

Robert Kay, M.D.
Cleveland Clinic Foundation
Cleveland, Ohio

M. Kathleen Kenyon
American Group Practice
 Association
Alexandria, Virginia

Jonna Kurucz
Prudential Insurance Company
Newark, New Jersey

Harold S. Luft
Institute for Health Policy
 Studies
San Francisco, California

Roice D. Luke
Virginia Commonwealth
 University
Richmond, Virginia

Douglas Mancino
Attorney
Los Angeles, California

Melinda McIntyre
Santa Monica Bank
Santa Monica, California

Gary Mendoza
Department of Corporations
Sacramento, California

Keith Moore
Consultant
Denver, Colorado

Thomas Morris, M.D.
School of Medicine, Columbia
  University
New York, New York

Cathy Murphy
Aetna Insurance
Hartford, Connecticut

Len Nichols
Urban Institute
Washington, D.C.

SallyAnne Payton
School of Law, University of
  Michigan
Ann Arbor, Michigan

Don Peck
The Advisory Board Company
Washington, D.C.

Patricia Powers
Pacific Business Group on
  Health
San Francisco, California

Ellen Pryga
American Hospital Association
Washington, D.C.

James Reinertsen, M.D.
HealthSystem Minnesota
Minneapolis, Minnesota

James C. Robinson
School of Public Health,
  University of California
Berkeley, California

William Sage
Columbia University School
  of Law
New York, New York

Barry Scheur
Consultant
Newton, Massachusetts

Richard Schwartz
The Advisory Board Company
Washington, D.C.

Siska Shaw
The Advisory Board Company
Washington, D.C.

Stephen M. Shortell
Kellogg Graduate School of
  Management, Northwestern
  University
Evanston, Illinois

Jacque Sokolov, M.D.
Advanced Health Plans
  and Coastal Physician
  Group, Inc.
Los Angeles, California

Michael Sparer
School of Public Health,
    Columbia University
New York, New York

Charles W. Stellar
American Managed Care and
    Review Association
Washington, D.C.

James Tallon
United Hospital Fund
New York, New York

Nicole Tapay
National Association of Insur-
    ance Commissioners
Washington, D.C.

Robert Tranquada, M.D.
University of Southern Califor-
    nia School of Medicine
Los Angeles, California

Michael Treash
Ernst and Young
Washington, D.C.

Walter Unger
Consultant
Orange County, California

Chris Varrone
The Advisory Board Company
Washington, D.C.

Mark Waxman
Attorney
Los Angeles, California

Alan Weil
Department of Health
Denver, Colorado

Alan Zwerner
United Medical Group
    Association
Los Angeles, California

Bibliography

Aaron, H. J. "Thinking Straight About Medical Costs." *Health Affairs,* Winter 1994, *13*(5), 8–13.

Abelson, R. "The Doctor Networks Aren't Created Equal: In a Hot New Sector, It Helps to View Performance as Well as the Promise." *New York Times,* Nov. 26, 1995, p. 4.

American Hospital Association. *Hospital Statistics: The AHA Profile of United States Hospitals.* (1994–1995 ed.) Chicago: American Hospital Association, 1994.

Anders, G., and Winslow, R. "The HMO Trend: Big, Bigger, Biggest." *Wall Street Journal,* Mar. 30, 1995.

Andrulis, D., and others. "Public Hospitals and Health Reform." Paper given to author, Aug. 1994.

"Bad News About Medicare HMOs: Results of HHS Inspector General's Survey of 4,132 Enrollees in 45 HMOs." From *Modern Healthcare,* March 20, 1995.

Bailey, A. "Charities Win, Lose in Health Shuffle." *The Chronicle of Philanthropy,* Jun. 14, 1994.

Baker, L. C. *Can Managed Care Control Health Care Costs: Evidence from the Medicare Experience.* Washington, D.C.: National Institute for Health Care Management, 1995.

Barrett, P. M. "Justices Allow States' Overhaul of Health Care." *Wall Street Journal,* Apr. 27, 1995.

"The Battle for Cleveland." *Integrated Healthcare Report,* Sept. 1994, pp. 1–8.

Bierig, J. R. "Antitrust and Physician Involvement in Managed Care: Reform is Needed!" Paper presented to the Physician Payment Review Commission as a critique of a manuscript entitled "Antitrust and Physician Involvement in Managed Care: Is Reform Needed?" by Arthur N. Lerner, Jan. 1995.

"Big New Chain's Tenet: Project Image of Integrity." *Health Alliance Alert,* Mar. 10, 1995, *10*(5).

Blankenau, R. "Measuring Up: Congress Reconsiders Tax-Exemption Standards Under Reform." *Hospitals & Health Networks,* Jan. 5, 1994, pp. 14–15.

Bloch, R. E. "Antitrust and Health Care." Paper presented at the National Health Policy Forum workshop on Consolidation in the Health Care Marketplace and Antitrust Policy, George Washington University, Washington, D.C., Jan. 1995.

Blumenthal, D. "Health Care Restructuring and Clinical Practice: Effects of Market Reforms on Doctors and Their Patients." Paper presented at the Robert Wood Johnson Foundation invitational meeting, The New Competition: Dynamics Shaping the Health Care Market, Nov. 1995, Washington, D.C.

Boisture, R. A. "Health Reform Speeds Shift to Tax-Exempt Integrated Managed Care Plans." *HealthSpan*, May 1994, *11*(5), 3–20.

Bradsher, K. "As 1 Million Leave Ranks of Insured, Debate Heats Up: Medicaid Battle Looms." *New York Times*, Aug. 27, 1995, Sec. 1, pp. 1, 20.

Braid, M., Manard, B., and Carney, B. *States as Payers: Managed Care for Medicaid Populations.* The States and Private Sector: Leading Health Care Reform, No. 2. Washington, D.C.: National Institute for Health Care Management, 1995.

Burda, D. "Mergers Thrive Despite Wailing About Adversity." *Modern Healthcare*, Oct. 12, 1992, pp. 26–28, 30, 32.

Burda, D. "For-Profits, Not-For-Profits Reignite Battle." *Modern Healthcare*, May 8, 1994, pp. 28, 30.

Burda, D. "How Close Is Too Close in Hospital Partnerships?" *Modern Healthcare*, Apr. 17, 1995a, pp. 26–28, 30, 32–33.

Burda, D. "Tennessee For-Profits Lag in Care for Poor." *Modern Healthcare*, Apr. 24, 1995b, pp. 70, 72, 74.

Cain Brothers. "Focus on Joint Venture Arrangements: Can Investor-Owned and Not-for-Profit Hospitals Bridge Ownership Differences?" *Strategies in Capital Finance*, vol. 12. New York: Cain Brothers, 1995.

"Can Academic Health Centers Survive?" *Integrated Healthcare Report*, Feb. 1995.

Carneal, C., and Gallmetzer, M. "Blurred Boundaries: State Regulation of PHOs." *HMO Magazine*, July/Aug. 1995, pp. 21–24.

"Catholic Values Cloud Hospital Deals." *Medicine & Health Perspectives*, May 29, 1995, *49*(22).

Center for the Study of Services. *Consumers' Checkbook: Consumer Guide to Health Plans.* Washington, D.C.: Center for the Study of Services, 1995.

Christensen, S. *The Effects of Managed Care and Managed Competition.* CBO Memorandum. Washington, D.C.: Congressional Budget Office, 1995.

Coile, R. C., Jr. "Assessing Healthcare Market Trends and Capital Needs: 1996–2000." *Healthcare Financial Management*, Aug. 1995, pp. 60–65.

"Columbia Closes Deal for Second Catholic Hospital in Past Year." *Health Alliance Alert,* Mar. 10, 1995, *10*(5).

"The Competitive Edge: Industry Report and Market Analysis." *Healthcare Trends Report,* May 1995, p. 9.

Conference Participants (Addendum), Community Snapshots Conference, sponsored by the Center for Studying Health System Change as part of the Robert Wood Johnson Foundation's Health Tracking Initiative, Washington, D.C., Dec. 13–14, 1995.

"Consolidated Checklist Merger Creates Statewide Catholic Coverage in California." *Health Alliance Alert,* Mar. 24, 1995, *10*(6).

"Consumer Satisfaction, Marketing, and Liability Take New Spotlight in the 1990s." *Managed Care Outlook,* Special Report.

"Corporate Takeover? Investor-Owned Systems Are Flexing Their Financial Muscles to Gain Greater Market Share." *Hospitals & Health Networks,* Mar. 20, 1995, pp. 44, 46.

"Cost, Not Quality or Satisfaction, Drive HMO Purchasing Decisions." *Managed Care Outlook,* Jul. 14, 1995, p. 6.

Cunningham, R. "Republicans Inherit Quest for Answers on Health Costs." *Medicine & Health Perspectives,* May 22, 1995a.

Cunningham, R. "Managed Care Agnostics Question Savings Claims." *Medicine & Health Perspectives,* Aug. 21, 1995b, pp. 1–4.

Dallek, G., Jimenez, C., and Schwartz, M. *Consumer Protections in State HMO Laws.* vol. 1: *Analysis and Recommendations.* Los Angeles: Center for Health Care Rights, 1995.

Davis, K., Collins, K. S., and Morris, C. "Managed Care: Promise and Concerns." *Health Affairs,* Fall 1994, pp. 178–185.

"A Delicate Balancing Act." *Modern Healthcare,* Mar. 13, 1995, pp. 34–36, 48.

"Do HMOs Care for the Chronically Ill?" *Healthcare Trends Report,* June 1995, p. 11.

"Doctors Are Increasingly Sharing Risks With HMOs." *Managed Care Outlook,* Mar. 10, 1995, p. 4.

"Doctors Are Losing Lobbying Battle to HMOs." *Wall Street Journal,* May 15, 1995.

"Doctors Rate the Big HMOs." *Healthcare Trends Report,* Mar. 1995, p. 12.

"The Dynamics of Market Reform." *Integrated Healthcare Report,* Apr. 1994, pp. 1–13.

"East Meets West." *Integrated Healthcare Report,* June 1994, pp. 1–5.

Eckholm, E. "A Hospital Copes With the New Order." *New York Times,* Jan. 29, 1993, Sect. 3, p. 1.

"Employers Increasingly Turn to Carve-Out Firms, Survey Finds." *Managed Care Outlook,* June 2, 1995, p. 9.

"Employers Forming National Coalition to Buy HMO Coverage." *Medicine & Health,* May 15, 1995.

Epstein, A. "America's Teaching Hospitals in the Evolving Health Care System." *Journal of the American Medical Association,* Apr. 19, 1995a, *273*(15).

Epstein, A. "Performance Reports on Quality—Prototypes, Problems and Prospects." *New England Journal of Medicine,* Jul. 6, 1995b, pp. 57–61.

"ERISA Ruling Opens the Door to More State Flexibility: Taxes Could Pay for Care for the Poor." *State Initiatives in Health Care Reform,* no. 13. Washington, D.C.: Alpha Center, Jul./Aug. 1995, pp. 1–4.

Ernst & Young LLP. *Physician-Hospital Organizations: State Regulators Play Catch-up.* Washington, D.C.: Ernst & Young LLP, 1994.

Ernst & Young LLP. *Physician-Hospital Organizations: Profile 1995.* Washington, D.C.: Ernst & Young LLP, 1995.

Etheredge, L. *The Evolution of a New Paradigm: Competitive Purchasing of Health Care.* Paper presented at the Robert Wood Johnson Foundation invitational meeting The New Competition: Dynamics Shaping the Health Care Market, Nov. 1995a.

Etheredge, L. *Reengineering Medicare: From Bill-Paying Insurer to Accountable Purchaser.* Research Agenda Brief. Washington, D.C.: Health Insurance Reform Project, George Washington University, June 1995b.

"Federal Court Gives Thumbs Down to AWP Law, Citing ERISA." *Managed Care Outlook,* May 19, 1995, p. 6.

Fein, E. "More Young Doctors Forsake Specialty for General Practice." *New York Times,* Oct. 16, 1995.

Fisher, I., and Fein, E. "Forced Marriage of Medicaid and Managed Care Hits Snags." *New York Times,* Aug. 28, 1995.

Foster Higgins. *National Survey of Employer-Sponsored Health Plans.* (10th ed.) New York: Foster Higgins, 1996.

Frazier, I. "The 'Care' in Health Care Reform: What Can States Do to Reform the Delivery System?" *State Health Care Reform,* vol. 1, no. 3. Washington, D.C.: Intergovernmental Health Policy Project, George Washington University, Aug. 1994.

Freudenheim, M. "Making Health Plans Prove Their Worth: A Lot Is Riding on a Pilot Program Comparing H.M.O.'s on Care and Cost." *New York Times,* Aug. 8, 1993.

Freudenheim, M. "Hospitals' New Creed: Less Is Best—No Areas Immune From Cost-Cutting." *New York Times,* Nov. 29, 1994, pp. D1, D17.

Freudenheim, M. "Business May Pay More for Health as Congress Cuts: Shift of Costs Expected." *New York Times,* Nov. 4, 1995a, sec. 1, pp. 1, 49.

Freudenheim, M. "Doctors, on Offensive, Form H.M.O.'s." *New York Times,* Mar. 7, 1995b.

Freudenheim, M. "Hospitals Are Tempted But Wary As For-Profit Chains Woo Them." *New York Times,* Jan. 4, 1995c, pp. A1, D5.

Freudenheim, M. "The New Breed of Insurance: Employers See Long-Term Savings in Hybrid Plans." *New York Times,* Jul. 28, 1995d.

Freudenheim, M. "As Blue Cross Plans Seek Profit, States Ask a Share of the Riches." *New York Times,* March 25, 1996.

"Friendly Hills Sold to CareMark: A Major Coup for CareMark." *Integrated Healthcare Report,* July 1994, pp. 8–9.

Fubini, S. "The Pace of Integration of Health Care." *Healthcare Trends Report,* Mar. 1995, *9*(3), 1, 15–16.

Fubini, S., and Antonelli, V. "1996 Industry Outlook." *Healthcare Trends Report,* Jan. 1996.

Gabel, J. R., and others. *HMO Industry Profile.* Washington, D.C.: Group Health Association, 1994.

Garvin, M. M., Ruger, T. W., and Roble, D. T. "Present and Future Strategies in the Managed Care Industry." Paper prepared for Ropes & Gray, Boston, Aug. 1994.

Gesensway, D. "Can PHOs Deliver On Their Promise?" *ACP Observer,* Dec. 1994, *14*(11), 1, 12–13.

Ginsburg, P. B. "Dynamics of Competition in Health Care: Overview." Paper presented at the Robert Wood Johnson Foundation invitational meeting The New Competition: Dynamics Shaping the Health Care Market, Washington, D.C., Nov. 1995.

Gold, M., and Camerlo, K. *Patterns in HMO Enrollment.* Washington, D.C.: Group Health Association of America, 1991.

Gold, M., and others. *Arrangements Between Managed Care Plans and Physicians: Results from a 1994 Survey of Managed Care Plans.* Selected External Research Series No. 3. Prepared under Grant #93–G08 to Mathematica Policy Research, Washington, D.C., and Medical College of Virginia, Richmond. Washington, D.C.: Physician Payment Review Commission, 1995.

Goldfarb, B. "Corporate Healthcare Mergers: Integrated Systems Between Private Companies, Hospitals and Large Group Practices May Dramatically Alter the Medical Landscape." *Medical World News,* Feb. 1993, pp. 26–28, 31–32, 34.

Goldsmith, J. C. "Driving the Nitroglycerin Truck." *Healthcare Forum Journal,* Mar./Apr. 1993a, pp. 36–38, 40, 44.

Goldsmith, J. C. "Hospital/Physician Relationships: A Constraint to Health Reform." *Health Affairs,* Fall 1993b, pp. 160–169.

Goldstein, A. "Medicaid Plan Calls for More Managed Care: Medicaid Would Save Half of Projected U.S. Cut." *Washington Post*, Oct. 12, 1995.

Gottlieb, M. "Picking a Health Plan: A Shot in the Dark." *New York Times*, Jan. 14, 1996, sec. 3, pp. 1, 9.

Governance Committee. *The Grand Alliance: Vertical Integration Strategies for Physicians and Health Systems.* Washington, D.C.: Advisory Board, 1993.

Governance Committee. *Grand Alliance II: Capitation Strategy.* Washington, D.C.: Advisory Board, 1994.

Governance Committee. *To the Greater Good: Recovering the American Physician Enterprise.* Washington, D.C.: Advisory Board, 1995.

Gray, B. Interview, 1995.

Greene, J. "Are Foundations Bearing Fruit?—Millions of Dollars are Doled Out for Research and Charity, But Critics Question the Community Benefit." *Modern Healthcare*, Mar. 20, 1995, pp. 53, 57–58, 68.

Greene, J., and Lutz, S. "Systems Post 4th Straight Year of Income Growth: Last Year's Merger Mania, Aggressive Cost Cutting Affect the Bottom Line, Annual Multi-Unit Providers Survey Shows." *Modern Healthcare*, May 23, 1994, pp. 36–38, 40, 42, 44, 46, 48–50, 52, 54, 56–58, 60, 62, 64–66, 68–70, 72–74, 76, 78, 80–82, 84–86, 88–92.

Greene, J., and Lutz, S. "A Down Year at Not-For-Profits: For-Profits Soar." *Modern Healthcare*, May 22, 1995, pp. 43–46.

Group Health Association of America. *Patterns in HMO Enrollment.* (2nd ed.) Washington, D.C.: Group Health Association of America, 1992.

Group Health Association of America. *Patterns in HMO Enrollment.* (4th ed.) Washington, D.C.: Group Health Association of America, 1995a.

Group Health Association of America. *HMO Fact Sheet.* Washington, D.C.: Group Health Association of America, 1995b.

Hagland, M. M. "Merger Mania? The Managed Care Field Consolidates—But Bigger Isn't Always Better." *Hospitals & Health Networks*, May 20, 1994, pp. 46–48, 50.

Havilecek, P. L., Eiler, M. A., and Neblett, O. T. *Medical Groups in the U.S.: A Survey of Practice Characteristics.* (1993 ed.) Chicago: American Medical Association, 1992.

Havilecek, P. L., Eiler, M. A., and Neblett, O. T. *Medical Groups in the U.S.: A Survey of Practice Characteristics.* (1996 ed.) Chicago: American Medical Association, 1995, Executive Summary.

"HCFA POS Guidelines Stalled as HMO Industry Cites Concerns." *Managed Care Outlook*, June 16, 1995, p. 4.

"Health Benefits in 1994." *Healthcare Trends Report*, Feb. 1995.

Health Care Advisory Board. *Line of Fire: The Coming Public Scrutiny of Hospital and Health System Quality.* Washington, D.C.: Advisory Board, 1993.

Health Care Advisory Board. *Network Advantage: Scale Economies and Cost Savings.* Washington, D.C.: Advisory Board, 1994.

Health Information Resources Group. *Hospital Closures, 1980–1993: A Statistical Profile.* Chicago: American Hospital Association, 1994.

"Health Plans Force Changes in the Way Doctors and Hospitals Are Paid." *New York Times,* Feb. 9, 1995, pp. A1, D5.

Healthcare Trends Report, Dec. 1995.

Hellinger, F. J. *Managing "Managed Care": The Expanding Scope of State Legislation.* Unpublished paper. Rockville, Md.: Agency for Health Care Policy and Research, Nov. 1995.

Hilzenrath, D. S. "Major HMO Operator Denied Accreditation: Mid Atlantic Medical Services Fails Rating." *Washington Post,* June 15, 1995, pp. B10, B12.

"HMOs Turn to Carve-Out Firms." *Managed Care Outlook,* June 2, 1995, p. 9.

Hodapp, T. E., and Samols, M. *HMOs 1995: The Right Place, the Right Time, the Right Idea.* San Francisco: Robertson, Stephens, 1994.

Holahan, J., and Liska, D. *The Impact of a Five Percent Medicaid Expenditure Growth Cap: A State Level Analysis.* Policy Brief. Washington, D.C.: Kaiser Commission on the Future of Medicaid, Kaiser Family Foundation, Mar. 1995.

"How Can Hospitals Survive?" *Hospital Management Review,* Oct. 1994, *13*(9), 1.

"How Close Is Too Close in Hospital Partnerships?" *Modern Healthcare,* April 17, 1995.

Jaklevic, M. "Docs Try to Own Managed Care." *Modern Healthcare,* Apr. 24, 1995.

Jensen, G. Untitled paper on Small Group Reforms presented to Alpha Center Conference, Robert Wood Johnson Foundation, Washington, D.C., Mar. 1995.

"Kaiser, Looking to Grow, Is Contracting with More Providers." *Managed Care Outlook,* May 19, 1995, p. 5.

Kertesz, L. "Managed-Care Contracts Up, But Capitation Hits Just 40 percent of California Providers—Study." *Modern Healthcare,* Apr. 24, 1995, p. 28.

Kertesz, L., and Wojcik, J. "Risky PHOs Winning Bet: Some Integrated Delivery Systems Are Pulling the Strings Under Capitation, But Many Will Find It Too Big a Gamble." *Modern Healthcare,* July 25, 1994, pp. 45–46, 48.

Koppelman, J. *Exploring the Impact of Medicaid Block Grants and Spending Caps.* National Health Policy Forum Issue Brief No. 660. Washington, D.C.: National Health Policy Forum, George Washington University, 1995.

Kralewski, J. "Consolidation of the Health Care Marketplace and Anti-Trust Policy: The Minnesota Experience." Paper presented at the National Health Policy Forum workshop on Consolidation in the Health Care Marketplace and Antitrust Policy, George Washington University, Jan. 1995.

Levitt, K., and others. "Home Health Care Expenditures, 1960–93." *Health Care Financing Review,* Fall 1994.

Luke, R. D., and Olden, P. C. "Foundations of Market Restructuring: Local Hospital Cluster and HMO Infiltration." *Medical Interface,* Sept. 1995, pp. 71–75.

Luke, R. D., Ozcan, Y. A., and Olden, P. C. *Local Markets and Systems: Hospital Consolidations in Metropolitan Areas.* Richmond: Department of Health Administration, Virginia Commonwealth University, Medical College of Virginia, 1995.

Lutz, S. "Let's Make a Deal: Healthcare Mergers, Acquisitions Take Place at Dizzying Pace." *Modern Healthcare,* Dec. 19–26, 1994, pp. 47–52.

Lutz, S. "The Question: Who's In Columbia/HCA's Sights?" *Modern Healthcare,* Jan. 2, 1995, p. 36.

Lutz, S. "Local Climates Drive Sales to Investor-Owned Chains." *Modern Healthcare,* Mar. 20, 1995, pp. 54, 56.

Managed Care Outlook, April 7, 1995, *8*(7), 2.

McCormick, B. "Courts Shaping Reform: Lawyers See Legal, Regulatory Actions Steering Market." *American Medical News,* June 26, 1995, pp. 1, 23.

"Medicare HMOs: Patient Satisfaction." *Health Care Financing Review,* 1993, *15*(1), 7.

"Medicare Risk Contracts Reach New Record High, HCFA Says." *Managed Care Outlook,* June 16, 1995, p. 3.

"Medpartners & Mullikin to Merge." *Integrated Healthcare Report,* July 1995, pp. 1–5.

Meyer, J., and others. *The Evolution of Managed Care: A Comparative Regional Analysis.* Washington, D.C.: New Directions for Policy, 1994.

"Mid-Sized Firms Embrace MCOs." *Managed Care Outlook,* Aug. 25, 1995, p. 8.

Miller, R. H., and Luft, H. S. "Managed Care: Past Evidence and Potential Trends." *Frontiers in Health Services Management,* 1993, *9*(3), 3–37.

Mitka, M. "HMOs See Steady Growth, Some Market Shifts." *American Medical News,* May 1, 1995, p. 9.

Morrisey, M., Jensen, G., and Morlock, R. "Data Watch: Small Employers and the Health Insurance Market." *Health Affairs,* Winter 1994, *13*(5), 149–161.

Murata, S. K. "Merger Mania: This Is the Year It Will Reach You." *Medical Economics,* Mar. 7, 1994, pp. 29–31, 33, 36.

"NAIC Guidelines Could Level Playing Field for Health Plans." *Managed Care Outlook*, Aug. 25, 1995, p. 3.

National Association of Insurance Commissioners. Memorandum to All Commissioners, Directors, and Superintendents: "Suggested Bulletin Regarding Certain Types of Compensation and Reimbursement Arrangements Between Health Care Providers and Individuals, Employers and Other Groups," Aug. 10, 1995.

National Committee for Quality Assurance. *Executive Summary for Report Card Pilot Project: Key Findings and Lessons Learned; Summary Performance Profile.* Washington, D.C.: National Committee for Quality Assurance, 1995a.

National Committee for Quality Assurance. *Medicaid HEDIS Executive Summary.* (Abbreviated summary of Medicaid HEDIS draft.) Washington, D.C.: National Committee for Quality Assurance, 1995b.

Neville, S. "Arizona's Managed Care System Offers Lessons for Rest of U.S." *Washington Post*, Sept. 25, 1995.

Nichols, L., and others. "Assessing Health System Integration: Lessons for State Policy Makers." Apr. 1995.

Noble, H. "Credit Agency Says Hospitals Face Hazards from Proposed Cuts." *New York Times*, Nov. 3, 1995.

"The Number of Americans With Health Insurance Coverage Continues to Drop." *State Initiatives in Health Care Reform*, No. 11. Washington, D.C.: Alpha Center, Mar./Apr. 1995, pp. 1–3.

Office of the General Counsel. *Antitrust: General Principles.* Q & A Report. Chicago: American Hospital Association, 1992.

Office of Technology Assessment. *Managed Care and Competitive Health Care Markets: The Twin Cities Experience.* Background Paper. Washington, D.C.: Government Printing Office, 1994.

Olmos, D. R. "UCLA, Santa Monica Hospitals to Merge." *Los Angeles Times*, 1995, pp. D1, D4.

"One-Quarter of U.S. Markets Have HMO Penetration of 25 percent." *Managed Care Outlook*, June 2, 1995, p. 3.

O'Sullivan, M. *Blue Cross' $2.5 Billion Grab: A Report on How Blue Cross of California Captured Billions of Dollars Owed to Health Charities.* San Francisco: Consumers Union, 1994.

Palzbo, S., and others. *HMO Industry Profile.* Washington, D.C.: Group Health Association of America, 1993.

Pear, R. "Florida Struggles to Lift Medicaid Burden." *New York Times*, Apr. 24, 1995.

Perrone, C., and Manard, B. *States as Purchasers: Innovations in State Employee Health Benefit Programs.* The States and Private Sector: Leading Health Care Reform, No. 3. Washington, D.C.: National Institute for Health Care Management, 1995. [Prepared by Lewin-VHI, Inc., April 1995]

Physician Payment Review Commission. *Annual Report to Congress 1995.* Washington, D.C.: Physician Payment Review Commission, 1995.

"Plans Pay Doctors Quality Bonuses to End Alienation, Improve Marketing." *Managed Care Week,* Supplement, Jan. 30, 1995, pp. 1–3.

Pogue, J. F. "Capitation Strategies." *Integrated Healthcare Report,* Dec. 1994, pp. 1–10.

Polzer, K. *Consolidation in the Health Care Marketplace and Antitrust Policy.* National Health Policy Forum Issue Brief No. 660. Washington, D.C.: National Health Policy Forum, George Washington University, n.d. (Advance publicity for conference held Jan. 17, 1995.)

"Purchasers Don't View NCQA Accreditation as Important." *Managed Care Outlook,* Aug. 25, 1995, p. 6.

"The Race to Consolidate." *Integrated Healthcare Report,* Mar. 1995.

Rich, S. "Medicaid's Safety Net for Children Could Be Imperiled, Reports Warn: Changes May Cut Coverage to Some If Parents Lose Private Insurance." *Washington Post,* Nov. 8, 1995.

Robert Wood Johnson Foundation. *Health Tracking: A Robert Wood Johnson Foundation Project Monitoring Health System Change.* Princeton, N.J.: Robert Wood Johnson Foundation, 1995. (Promotional folder containing brochure on Center for Studying Health System Change, brochure on Health Tracking Project, and Community Snapshots factsheets.)

Robinson, J. C. "Organizational Re-Alignment in Competitive Medical Markets." Paper presented at the Robert Wood Johnson Foundation invitational meeting The New Competition: Dynamics Shaping the Health Care Market, Washington, D.C., Nov. 1995.

Robinson, J. C., and Casalino, L. P. "The Growth of Medical Groups Paid Through Capitation in California." *New England Journal of Medicine,* Dec. 21, 1995, *333*(25), 1684–1687.

Rosenbaum, S. Paper presented at U.S. Department of Health and Human Services conference, 1995.

Rosenthal, E. "New York Faults H.M.O.'s for Poor Service: A Plan for Regulation—State Will Require Standards for Better Service and for Greater Accountability." *New York Times,* Nov. 17, 1995, pp. A1, B4.

Rowland, D., and others. "Medicaid and Managed Care: Lessons from the Literature." Prepared for the Kaiser Commission on the Future of Medicaid, Nov. 1994.

Rundle, R. L. "Big Charities Born as Health Plans Go For Profit." *Wall Street Journal,* Apr. 4, 1995a.

Rundle, R. L. "Observers Detect a Health-Care Giant Looming in Well-Point-Health Systems." *Wall Street Journal,* Apr. 4, 1995b.

Sack, K. "Public Hospitals Around the Country Cut Basic Service," *New York Times,* Aug. 20, 1995.

Samuelson, R. J. "Managed-Care Revolution." *Washington Post,* Oct. 25, 1995.

Sardinha, C. "MCOs Scramble to Cut Hospital Usage as LOS Rates Hit New Lows." *Managed Care Outlook,* Jan. 13, 1995a, *8*(1), 1–3.

Sardinha, C. "Integrated Delivery Systems Come Under Fire from Plans, Employers." *Managed Care Outlook,* Mar. 24, 1995b, *8*(6), 1–3.

Sardinha, C. "Firms Launch National Purchasing Coalition, But HMOs Growing Weary." *Managed Care Outlook,* June 2, 1995c, *8*(11), 1–3.

Serafini, M. W. "Not So Fast." *National Journal,* Dec. 17, 1994, pp. 2967–2970.

Service, M. "Why Health Costs Got Smaller in 1994." *Business & Health,* March 1995, pp. 20–28.

Shactman, D., and Altman, S. H. *Market Consolidation, Antitrust, and Public Policy in the Health Care Industry: Agenda for Future Research.* Waltham, Mass.: Council on the Economic Impact of Health Care Reform, Institute for Health Policy, The Heller School, Brandeis University, Feb. 1995.

Shipley, K. "Suggested Bulletin Regarding Certain Types of Compensation and Reimbursement Arrangements Between Health Care Providers and Individuals, Employers and Other Groups." *Memorandum to All Commissioners, Directors, and Superintendents.* (pp. 1–8) Alexandria, Va.: National Association of Insurance Commissions, 1995.

Shortell, S. M., Gillies, R. R., and Anderson, D. A. "New World of Managed Care: Creating Organized Delivery Systems." *Health Affairs,* Winter 1994, *13*(5), 46–64.

Shortell, S. M., and Hull, K. E. *The New Organization of Health Care: The Evolution of Managed Care and Delivery Systems.* Paper prepared for Baxter II Health Policy Review. Evanston, Ill.: J. L. Kellogg Graduate School of Management, Northwestern University, Oct. 1994.

Shriver, K. "Study: Most Hospitals Will Try Integration Despite Obstacles." *Modern Healthcare,* Dec. 12, 1994, p. 4.

"Sick People in Managed Care Have Difficulty Getting Services and Treatment, New Survey Reports." *Healthcare Trends Report,* July 1995, p. 8.

Slomski, A. J. "Hospitals' Little Secret: They Make Lots of Money." *Medical Economics,* Mar. 27, 1995, pp. 66–68, 73–74.

Solovy, A. "Predicting the Unpredictable." *Hospitals & Health Networks,* Jan. 5, 1995, *69*(1), 26.

"Stephen M. Shortell, Ph.D.: The Future of Integrated Systems." (Interview) *Healthcare Financial Management,* Jan. 1995, pp. 24–26, 28.

Steptoe, M. L. "Current Issues in Health Care Antitrust: Boycotts, Mergers, and Provider Networks." Prepared remarks presented before the American Bar Association Section of Antitrust Law Spring Meeting, Washington, D.C., Apr. 1995.

Swartz, K., and Brennan, T. A. "Integrated Health Care, Capitated Payment and Quality: The Role of Regulation." *Annals of Internal Medicine,* Feb. 15, 1996.

Terry, K. "Look Who's Guarding the Gate to Specialty Care." *Medical Economics,* Aug. 22, 1994a, pp. 124–132.

Terry, K. "HMO Deals That Give You More Money for More Risk." *Medical Economics,* Dec. 26, 1994b, pp. 30–33, 37–38, 40.

Terry, K. "Has Managed Care Rediscovered Fee-For-Service?" *Medical Economics,* July 10, 1995, pp. 69–70, 75–76, 79–80.

Thornburg, A. M. "Financial Implications and Management Challenges of the New Health Alliances and Integrated Delivery Systems." Presentation at Harvard Conference on Strategic Alliances in the Evolving Healthcare Market, Boston, Nov. 3, 1995.

Tokarski, C. "A Nonprofit or For-Profit Health System: Does It Matter?" *Medicine & Health Perspectives,* Feb. 7, 1994.

Tokarski, C. "A New Rhythm for the Blues." *Hospitals & Health Networks,* Mar. 5, 1995, *69*(5), 23–26.

Walker, L. "How Big Is Doctor's Prepaid Income?" *Medical Economics,* Oct. 23, 1995, *72*(20), 172–182.

"Warning Signs on the Road to Managed Care." *Commonwealth Fund Quarterly,* Summer 1995, *1*(2), 1–2.

Whitener, M. D. "Antitrust, Medicare Reform and Health Care Competition." Prepared remarks before the American Enterprise Institute for Public Policy Research, Washington, D.C., Dec. 1995.

Winslow, R. "Medical Upheaval: Welfare Recipients Are a Hot Commodity in Managed Care Now." *Wall Street Journal,* Apr. 12, 1995.

Zeckhauser, R. J. "Game Theory Insights for Hospital Alliance Decisions." Paper presented at Harvard Conference on Strategic Alliances in the Evolving Healthcare Market, Boston, Dec. 2, 1995.

Zwanziger, J. "The Need for an Antitrust Policy for a Health Care Industry in Transition." *Journal of Health, Politics, Policy, and Law,* 1995a, *20*(1), 171–173.

Zwanziger, J. "The Effect of Price Competition on Health Care Costs." Paper presented at the Robert Wood Johnson Foundation invitational meeting The New Competition: Dynamics Shaping the Health Care Market, Washington, D.C., Nov. 1995b.

Index